I0568515

Grief

Recovery

A Guide to Recovery From Grief and Loss of a Loved One

(Grief Recovery Method for Healing Through the Different Stages of Grief)

Johnnie Logan

Published By **Jordan Levy**

Johnnie Logan

All Rights Reserved

Grief Recovery: A Guide to Recovery From Grief and Loss of a Loved One (Grief Recovery Method for Healing Through the Different Stages of Grief)

ISBN 978-1-998769-85-8

No part of this guidebook shall be reproduced in any form without permission in writing from the publisher except in the case of brief quotations embodied in critical articles or reviews.

Legal & Disclaimer

The information contained in this ebook is not designed to replace or take the place of any form of medicine or professional medical advice. The information in this ebook has been provided for educational & entertainment purposes only.

The information contained in this book has been compiled from sources deemed reliable, and it is accurate to the best of the Author's knowledge; however, the Author cannot guarantee its accuracy and validity and cannot be held liable for any errors or omissions. Changes are periodically made to this book. You must consult your doctor or get professional medical advice before using any of the suggested remedies, techniques, or information in this book.

Upon using the information contained in this book, you agree to hold harmless the Author from and against any damages, costs, and expenses, including any legal fees potentially resulting from the application of any of the information provided by this guide. This disclaimer applies to any damages or injury caused by the use and application, whether directly or indirectly, of any advice or information presented, whether for breach of contract, tort, negligence, personal injury, criminal intent, or under any other cause of action.

You agree to accept all risks of using the information presented inside this book. You need to consult a professional medical practitioner in order to ensure you are both able and healthy enough to participate in this program.

Table Of Contents

Chapter 1: Coping With Grief

Experiencing grief is human nature and is a standard reaction whilst losing a person close to you. The way humans grieve is particular from each other; however, the system involved is the identical in dropping a person expensive to you, ending a dating from a person vast for your existence, if you are recognized with an ailment, losing your home or your source of profits, and other horrible losses. The severity of 1's grief is definitely associated with the intensity of the character's regard to the individual or assets that became misplaced.

Telling any other man or woman and expressing feelings regarding the loss is a tremendous factor so as for restoration to continue. Speak to every other person who is inclined to hear you out, is accepting of you, and does no longer make any attempt to make you feel in any other case. Sharing with some other individual or group of people can help in a single's undertaking to begin spotting and embracing the reality of his or her loss.

Recognition of emotions

Acknowledge that how someone feels or gets in contact together with his emotion is a part of life and is critical within the process of recuperation. Relate to the manner you sense, become aware of the emotion, and explicit it verbally or thru writing. Some be part of the theater to act out their feelings, while others either dance or sing. People have numerous alternatives that suit their desires in managing grief and save you to be overwhelmed with the aid of the surge of ache and other difficult emotions that can arise. The profoundness of these feelings could make a person experience rebellious, defiant, or unmanageable. These strong feelings can conquer own coping skills. Grief is much like the climate. Sometimes it's far like mere drops of rain and at times it is available in torrents.

Acceptance of grief

Appropriateness in managing grief and the way humans grieve may additionally vary. One thing to keep in mind is not to submerge or keep it locked inside. It is likewise now not really helpful to elude such feelings. In order to efficaciously overcome it, grief needs to be diagnosed and embraced and let all of the feelings that include it to just flow evidently. Emotions associated with grieving fluctuate in every section. At the onset, the man or woman might also veer faraway from recognizing the loss. He can be in a nation of surprise, defiance, and resentment.

It can take months to be within the denial segment however in some months, the individual may begin to face up to the truth of his loss and can have more manipulate over his emotions of sorrow, rage, overwhelming distress, dread, self-blame, and depression. In the following year, he may additionally start to acknowledge his loss and receive this truth in his existence. Previous severe emotions will start to mild and he may additionally start to have feelings of bliss and peace of thoughts.

When you turn out to be aware about and communicate your feelings within the direction of the numerous levels of the grief process, bear in mind it isn't which you are experiencing an awful day, however a second of grief. Grief happens and it can't be stopped like nobody can forestall an coming near hurricane or the setting of the sun. You can handiest go along with the glide of your grief and find a stable and comforting vicinity to proportion it. It is imperative to give time to understand which you are hurting in the intervening time, due to the fact delaying it will handiest come back later on in life. Link with whom or what you lost, and after you are organized, make use of what are saved for your memory including pix, locations, clothes, and others to make you feel cared for and calm.

Phases of Grief

Every character goes through the numerous stages of grief in extraordinary methods. The technique can take as long as the man or woman needs. While they walk into this method, they'll get inside and outside of 1 segment extra than as soon as.

Avoidance

Distress, lack of feeling, defiance, and doubt are the first responses while a person grieves. He may additionally grow to be inundated with mind of being in an illusory or surreal country. This in most cases occurs with unanticipated loss. A person needs enough time for his disbelief to impede. Defiance and denial lets him recognize a few portions of his fact in a progressive manner. Disputing the loss and being enraged could occur once the person is out of shock or denial and starts offevolved to recognize the reality in his life. Usually, the man or woman asks outwardly why this occurred to him and why life isn't always fair to him. When someone feels out of control he is willing to are searching for out the solutions of unanswerable questions in his head. He may additionally experience chargeable for not being capable of prevent or save you what befell. In truth, there is no genuine solution and no one responsible. When the man or woman has exerted all his efforts thinking and appearing out his frustration and rage, he can also start to move directly to the subsequent phase.

Longing and in search of for what become lost is just one of the many methods to dispute the loss. It is commonplace for the man or woman at this moment to go through the activities or what happened earlier than the occasion passed off. He may additionally inform himself that he might not have revel in this devastating loss if he had accomplished some thing to save you it or if he made things different. These matters he expresses simplest reflect his very sturdy preference to have some control over the things that befell. But wallowing on those mind will now not assist him pass on.

Instead, he'll simply be moving into and out of that phase.

In this stage, the individual might imagine some thing incorrect befell along the way which caused his distressing loss. He may also choose to feel that matters can be the manner they have been and that character he loves will reappear in his existence or the activity he lost will nonetheless be looking forward to him at the office. He may additionally conquer those illogical mind within some months. Truth is that masses of humans undergo these feelings specially within the severe section of grieving. Usually round this time, the individual starts to get in and get out of the avoidance segment to get into the confrontation phase as he faces the reality in his life that what he misplaced will in no way come again.

Confrontation

This stage starts offevolved with being aware that his existence will now not be the way it had been. The person may additionally have long past beyond having surreal thoughts approximately his existence. He may additionally start acknowledging that his lifestyles at the prevailing time is his reality. At this moment, grief can be very profound. Any character can sense very sensitive which every now and then may be overpowering. This can result in a state of getting disorganized.

Rage-depression, desperation, despair-disappointment, overwhelming distress, terror, self-blame, and disorganization are common responses whilst the man or woman in grief has proven his first emotions of rage and frustration for his loss. These can come as bereavement starts offevolved. In his instance, accepting the ache is quite imperative. At this second also, anyone need to experience worn out and extraordinarily miserable. The excessive weariness, problem focusing, hassle with slumbering or oversleeping, and feelings of intense vulnerability are all standard for a person who is utterly depressed and grieving. It won't be that difficult to tell others you feel overly depressed. It is greater beneficial to claim this adverse however reflective moment of your existence as melancholic and grief. Medical practitioners can provide an explanation for if a person's disappointment and grief have turn out to be depression. A a part of each of those areas is a sense of despondency with the know-how that traditional beliefs had been disconcerted.

There is ache, desolation, and a certain great to every area or phase. The experience of order and thinking of his personal world by an individual experiencing grief has been affected. Consequently, his lifestyles will no longer be the same as he knew it. He may additionally sense enraged that a person or different things pricey to him are all the time gone. To the volume that he may additionally sense a exquisite a part of his being has additionally died. With this kind of loss, momentarily he may think that nothing has been left for him to head on with existence.

It is also viable that he becomes mystified of who he absolutely is, his position, and what truly manner to him.

Generally, humans choose to be on top of things in their lives. If a few tragedy or event happens that makes a person lose manage, he can also develop an illogical reasoning that he had permit down the standards society dictated, with himself protected. Depression or depression in this phase may want to end result to the individual feeling he's going to not be capable of revel in happiness on this lifetime. This is an ordinary feeling for folks that are heartbroken. Grief brings out feelings which include dread, anger, guilt, and despair. Feeling each emotion is a herbal crucial process. Sadness is an possibility to preserve things slow and be reflective. It is with the aid of mirrored image and reassessment of one's lifestyles that gaining knowledge of and the capacity to move on can take place. Due to severe hurtfulness and desperation, the individual may expect for different human beings to mend the damaged pieces, provide comfort, and make the matters that reason him grief to disappear. Grief is a unique technique and it's far tough additionally for the individuals who are inside the identical way convoluted with disappointment to attain for you and provide comfort. People ought to keep in thoughts that grief isn't always some thing that can be managed and shortened. Every individual has a completely unique length of grieving time so he can take the subsequent step and circulate on together with his lifestyles.

Accommodation

A character may additionally slowly get into this segment considering that feelings concerned in grief are step by step diminishing and social and emotional connection with daily dwelling is beginning. The character begins to live his existence after the loss without needing to keep away from its fact. This method he has already established the loss and the adjustments in his lifestyles that go along with such event. With the dying of a loved one, which means he's now reconnecting with this character in a different way. If he have become sick and misplaced his youthful health, in the accommodation phase he has emerge as accepting of his condition and makes the maximum out of his existence and current condition.

The initiation and place to begin of reorganization show up simplest after the craze, sadness, and depression were shown. The person wishes to permit go of these emotions however no longer the connection with the man or woman he lost. The courting will constantly be there in spite of the hurt and sadness. This phase won't be smooth and may only show up in little steps. The day will come whilst the notion of getting misplaced that special individual becomes tolerable or presents an opportunity to stop being unhappy and distressed. The look for significance in life begins that's a robust indicator that the character is beginning to heal.

Acceptance, popularity, and reorganization display that the person has end up conscious he has no different choice but to prepare himself of the truth that his dating with the person he misplaced has changed. His search for significance and reorganizing his lifestyles becomes especially vital in this segment of grief.

Chapter 2: Navigating Thru Grief

Some human beings might imagine that grief is inculcated with inconsistencies. People are expected to express their goodbyes and yet devise way to keep connections through pictures and different memoirs of human beings with whom these connections have passed on. People usually find method to provide regard to the lives of folks that passed; however, grief is all approximately those who've been left behind. It is a second of reputation with the termination of a courting or occupation and is about new beginnings in existence. The standard technique of grieving has various stages and can occur bodily, via emotional suffering, or irrational mind and moves. At the equal time as grief includes essential characteristics, each passage is distinct. Many surprise the way to navigate thru this puzzling maze of grief. There are fundamental methods to perform this:

• Give yourself time to experience the pain of loss – Feelings are available in all types and at diverse times. Some may additionally feel at peace however then may additionally explicit their emotions via crying and feeling sad. Others may additionally shed tears without know-how what had prompt this burst of emotion. There may be uncertainty, melancholy, rage, tiredness, marvelous clearness, resilience, either beneath-consuming or overeating and sound asleep issues, unexpected interest with the aid of pals who are not that near, overpowering affection, fear, flashbacks, self-blame, discomfort, and disappointment for lost possibilities. These are matters that want to be felt and shared or expressed.

• Express self thru ritual - A lot of feelings are manifested even more via ritual. Find approach considerable to you that offer console on the same time incite inscrutability. Some of those rituals may contain quiet time, song, sizeable private gadgets, poetry, lighting up a candle, and other easy movements. The concepts may additionally have variations inclusive of rituals for being free from attachments, rituals for unique kinds of memoirs, or showing forgiveness.

• Have a break – There is nothing more momentous and earth-shattering than the start as well as the passing of a loved one. The feeling of loss might also haunt you for some time, and for a few this can move on even for years. However, it gets much less and much less tough in time. There are numerous elements which can effect the passage of bereavement. These encompass the period of the connection, the participation of the individual on your lifestyles, and his importance to you and the people around. If there has been distress within the direction of courting or the scenario surrounding the death, emotional feelings are greater and more extreme. It can be loads superb to navigate via a complex grief adventure with a professional or a therapist. Sometimes only expert practitioners can point out what is essentially the trouble when all coping capabilities had been executed and the character remains distant, disorganized, and not able to decide his destiny.

• Make connections with the residing – Grief may be a herbal a part of being human but it is able to be more difficult than it's miles perceived. It is notably beneficial to percentage emotions and thoughts to individuals who are enduring the equal ache and going via similar adventure. They can attain support and external strength from a pool of know-how and reviews others are inclined to proportion. Nowadays, plenty of humans locate solace in achieving to others via way of worldwide interconnectivity, group support activities, and cyber boards.

Grief and Mindfulness

Mindfulness is a perception extensively held amongst persons who exercise Buddhism. It is profoundly connected to the concept of impermanence. If someone regards or believes inside the idea of impermanence, he can either start to assume what's in keep for him in the future fixatedly or he can also live constantly inside the beyond. Acceptance of impermanence basically manner dwelling at the existing.

Mindfulness is a way of dwelling through which a person turns into conscious of his truth, mind, emotions, and physical encounters inside the gift time. As he acknowledges that nothing is everlasting, he can perceive his life now and inspect what he without a doubt feels. The idea of meditation however is a way for humans to collect studying and apply mindfulness to day by day living understanding that not anything in this existence is everlasting.

Significance of mindfulness to grief

People deal with grief by using becoming totally crushed and absorbed by using their heartache or they keep away from ache and feelings for worry of having trapped in grief. As a result, they circulate on without grieving. With mindfulness, humans can comprehend that like the whole lot else, those negative feelings also are not everlasting. However, getting beyond grief isn't an immediate occurrence. It takes time and there are methods concerned people want to undergo. Acceptance of the realities of lifestyles which include loss and pain can facilitate in starting up the system of diminishing grief. People can begin no longer to consider it is going on all the time even supposing that is how they experience for the time being. They can begin taking be aware and embracing their grief for what it sincerely is as well as the little changes of their every day reports.

Implementing mindfulness

This meditation practice begins with respiration from the diaphragm and being conscious of every breath. This form of respiratory exercise expands the diaphragm as you inhale and settlement as you breathe out. Begin by using taking a seat with legs crossed, muscular tissues comfortable, and the frame very directly. Identify some thing in front you could attention on and maintain a comfortable function for the jaws, shoulders, and fingers. Make positive you are occupying a noiseless vicinity with out interruptions. When you are already relaxed however targeted, begin the respiratory and be counted each breath. At the onset, you could vicinity one hand in your stomach to make certain your respiration remains within the diaphragm. Count each exhalation.

People should know that meditation isn't focused on clearing the thoughts definitely because this is subsequent to impossible. It is less complicated to understand and practice that meditation is absolutely approximately being privy to one's mind and letting them go. Once you begin respiratory, begin to focus on your frame motion, the motion of air, and preserve counting the wide variety of breaths. You want to maintain the counts and veer away from distractive mind. If some mind linger, simply recognize them and let them move. It can be amazing to be aware about how a great deal notion someone will have in such brief time from barking dogs, starvation pang or thirst, dripping tap, passing automobiles, the concept of what you lately misplaced, thoughts on what the destiny will carry, activities for the day, tomorrow, and the following day, amongst others. Initially, letting move of these styles of mind may be hard to accomplish. One thought ought to branch out to other mind and so on. You will not notice what's taking place, but you might be losing rely of your breaths and losing awareness on the pastime handy. This is hard to muster before everything, however with constant exercise, in the end you could get the hang of it. Some humans follow the "leaves on a stream" visualization method. This is explained step by step within the next bankruptcy.

This technique works by using now not permitting one's thoughts managed and avoid frightening mind. On the alternative hand, mindfulness instructs the man or woman to end up aware about his present day thoughts, accept them, and let them pass. While making use of mindfulness, its beneficial effects can extend to daily sports. While a person runs through his activities of every day life which may be very difficult to do inside the system of grief, mindfulness may be integrated step by step. He may be conscious of his thoughts, take note of them, embody and understand them, then let them pass. At the identical time, he need to stay focused at the modern-day time and undertaking at hand.

For example, a person who currently lost loved ones like in a catastrophic event, he observed operating his automobile a tough challenge that he cannot do it without crying. This saved occurring for months. He would appear on top of things in different components of his life besides when starting his automobile. With mindfulness, he changed into capable of consciousness on his breathing at the same time as riding. This approach concentrating at the mechanical issue and physical enjoy of riding whilst he starts offevolved to sense inundated with bad emotions. He might deal with turning into aware of his mind and permitting them to move, concentrating again on his respiratory and driving. This is less complicated said than achieved but all things need to start somewhere. As time goes it becomes much less and less difficult and could afterward be part of the way he faces the world.

Chapter 3: Visualization Technique

There are other versions of the "leaves on a circulation" visualization approach. Visualize the picture of a move along the periphery of a wooded area. Whenever a notion involves thoughts simply notice it, perceive the idea, and make a intellectual image of it as a leaf drifting at the movement. Look on the leaf as it glides down the movement of water till it vanishes and then cross again to concentrating to your respiration.

• Imagine your self located along the threshold of the stream. Looking at the water slowly jogging. You also can make a intellectual photograph of yourself placed inside the midst of the circulate, staring at the water walking faraway from you.

• Hear the water whilst it flows. You can see a mental photo of the mild while it seeps via the leaves to move over the floor of the water.

- Take observe of the leaves that come from distinctive varieties of trees. They have diverse shapes, sizes, and colorings drifting at the water passing you by using or flowing away from you as the cutting-edge takes them farther away.

- Take heed of any feelings, feelings, or mind coming to you, whether they're high quality, negative, or neither. Put every thought on a leaf. Observe the leaf as it glides away, floating its manner toward the other a part of the flow.

- Sometimes, you may see your self perched on a leaf along with one of your thoughts or emotions. Let this take place. Let it retain and simply examine.

- Allow the stream to flow the way it wants to. If you feel you need to sluggish down or quicken the move's movement, you can positioned that impulse on a leaf like what you did with mind and emotions. Never attempt to manage this activity.

- If a leaf gets stuck inside the water, you just need to allow things go and have a look at what occurs. It is not necessary to do any movement toward it.

• Keep searching on the stream. If there are extra mind or feelings coming to you, just area each one on a leaf.

• Through certainly observing mind and emotions glide away, you could start to suppose that those mind and feelings aren't your self but best things you maintain directly to.

• Once you're organized, allow the picture of the jogging water to disappear. Bring your focus returned to the real international wherein you are.

•

Relaxation Techniques

People analyze and develop as they exert notable effort in managing their ache. Part of managing pain is handling one's thoughts. When you cope with those mind, it's far simpler to find forgiveness and find out what matters most to you. As the importance of existence for you offers a extraordinary meaning, you may begin to doubt the ideals and viewpoints you had. You experience the want to make huge modifications in existence like making the most of your time and doing more activities which might be useful to others and to the arena in general. Things you cherish formerly come to be less essential now. This may be wonderful for you however the individuals who care for you may study these changes in another way. So even as going thru positive lifestyles changes, it's miles imperative to verbalize the manner those changes are making effect to you and your life.

Relaxation strategies can be beneficial in case you are uneasy, tensed, and in case your time table is aggravating or you not realize a way to relax efficiently. While grieving, the situation may additionally seem overly self-absorbed to think of relaxing strategies for your self. But in case you are within the method of grief, your body is also under duress and if you do now not allow your self time to recharge and sluggish down or unwind there is a opportunity that you may increase physical ailments.

At first, effective relaxation strategies are great accomplished inside a time and vicinity without disturbances and constraints. With enough exercise and willpower, it is able to be clean to experience rest strategies. One of the most desired and effective relaxation methods is meditation. This may be very powerful and can be done at any vicinity and time. With those relaxation strategies, someone's chance to be psychologically or physically sick can be reduced. These techniques may be utilized to prepare self for a few meditation and be geared up to face humans and interact with them in different situations. Keep those techniques available. They can be beneficial when you experience your muscle tissues getting worrying and you are overworked or crushed with the stresses of life, or while your mind is extraordinarily occupied.

Choose rest techniques you could use whenever. Begin with the everyday techniques you already know or those which you continually use efficaciously. Add greater strategies so you can have an assortment of activities which are powerful for you. Some relaxation strategies are as follows:

• Meditation

• Mindful activities (via respiratory and meditation)

• Massage

• Walking

• Muscle rest or progressive muscle rest

• Tai Chi

• Yoga

• Pilates

• Running

Muscle Relaxation

There is a shape of muscle rest that can be used to meditate. It is focused on the physical issue of the body since the muscle groups can keep a whole lot of anxiety with the day by day stresses human beings face. The steps for this form of meditation are as follows:

• Lie down or sit down at ease with the body in a directly line. Open the chest with the shoulders returned and down. Eyes must be saved closed. Concentrate on breathing and take three smooth, lengthy, and deep breaths just like the respiratory techniques used within the Mindful respiration sporting activities.

• Keep recognition of your respiration whilst additionally focusing at the frame. Make use of respiration to disperse sore or tight areas of the frame.

• Concentrate at the feet and ft and notice if there may be any anxiety in those regions. Squeeze the feet and toe muscle groups then hold this for ten to twenty seconds.

• Make it a slow, lengthy, and gentle exhalation on your next breath. Let go of any anxiety in the ft and toes, and then loosen up. You can feel them soften as you complete this project.

• Focus now on the bottom and legs. If there may be any anxiety on those muscle tissue, constrict the muscular tissues for ten to twenty seconds.

• Make a gentle, slow, and long breath in your next breath. Let move of any anxiety inside the stomach and the bottom. Relax and you'll observe they have become smooth.

• Concentrate at the lower back, the chest, and shoulders. Squeeze the muscles in those regions for ten to 20 seconds making sure your chest is out, the lower back is directly, and the shoulders are returned and down. Relax until the muscle tissues grow to be gentle.

• Make your fingers straight at the side. Focus at the palms, palms, and the shoulders. Be privy to any tension in these regions. Close the fists firmly and squeeze the muscle tissues inside the arms, the fingers, and shoulders for ten to 20 seconds.

• Make a gradual, mild and lengthy exhalation and let pass of all tension that comes from the arms, palms, and shoulders. Relax and word how they become smooth after.

• Raise the shoulders as high as you can and preserve them for ten to 20 seconds, then decrease them and take the shoulders lower back and down. Relax till muscle tissues are absolutely softened.

• Concentrate now at the face, neck area, and the head. Squeeze the muscle mass to tighten and keep for ten to twenty seconds.

• Make the subsequent mild, lengthy, and slow exhalation and let pass of all the anxiety in the neck, face, and head regions. Relax until these regions sense soft.

• Slowly at the same time as exhaling circulate the head in the direction of the left. Let it stay that manner for five seconds and on the subsequent breath, bring the top in the direction of the middle.

• As you exhale, slowly pass the chin closer to the chest and permit it live for five seconds. On the next breath, deliver the head again to its former position or the center.

• Slowly as you exhale carry the chin and head up towards the again. Hold this role for 5 seconds. Bring the pinnacle back to the middle on the subsequent breath.

• Move the top in the direction of the left and preserve for 5 seconds. As you exhale, deliver the pinnacle to the center.

• Keep concentrating for your respiratory and make 3 clean, deep, and long breaths.

After a session of this muscle rest, you may experience your frame becoming light and is unfastened from anxiety. Set apart a couple of minutes of your day to exercise this rest technique.

Grief Meditation

It is ordinary for humans to instinctively communicate approximately past reports, having a mental picture of a near person they recently misplaced. This priceless internal association can be deliberately nurtured. Grief meditation is particularly fitting if the connection is primarily based on an affectionate dating.

Make time of at the least fifteen mins a day with out distractions and have your eyes closed. Begin with three minutes just concentrating to your personal respiration at tempo even as you're in a comfortable position. Let a visible imagery of a picturesque region enter your thoughts. It must be one that is serene and makes you at ease. While it arises to your mind, take note of the colors, sounds, smells, and textures. Notice the manner you experience approximately being in this non violent vicinity. In addition, take with you whatever into that place whatever a good way to toughen your comfortable nation. Enjoy this time whilst bringing in all of the advantageous emotions it invokes inside you.

After some time, you can name inside the individual you misplaced to come back to the location, being conscious that the individual's imagery may additionally are available in various forms and might come into sight at any age. Do no longer hurry and take all of the time you need to welcome him and tell him anything you want to mention. Encourage him to communicate to you. Let this come across expand on its very own encouraging a herbal connection at the equal time not going past your comfort sector.

Express your gratitude to this person for coming and sharing this time with you. Close your imagery imaginative and prescient whilst you take your self again to fact. Take time to truely feel your emotions and indulge inside the revel in you simply went via. Keep in mind that your conditions in life may work via adjustments and your emotions may additionally come and cross, to the quantity that you battle with looking for answers to questions which could by no means be replied. However, you continually want to be resilient, aspire to be stronger or extra strong, and not lose your self in something circumstance you discover yourself in.

Chapter 4: Self-Care Is Compulsory

Grief may be unpleasant, jarring, and nasty. You ought to take responsibility for your self whilst you are grieving. Self-care is essential to rehabilitation and enables lessen intellectual, bodily, and non secular ache. The manner that everybody offers with unhappiness and movements via the grieving procedure differs. It is okay if what labored for another character does now not give you the results you want.

Whenever each person near you passes away, everything can fast trade. In the start, you'll be capable of divert yourself through maintaining busy and looking after sensible subjects like funeral arrangements. The reality of the loss can finally sink in, causing you to fear about how you'll cope, perhaps following the funeral, for instance, whilst your lifestyles seems to return to "everyday."

Every man or woman expresses grief in another way. Our awesome grieving trips are on the whole shaped with the aid of the specific traits we each possess. There are different different styles of loss as well, consisting of a liked one to demise, separation, a courting breakdown, a terminal ailment, drug utilization, and so forth. Some humans suddenly revel in loss. Some humans had expected it.

This feeling is difficult regardless of how you ended up inside the trenches of loss. And then, whilst we strive to bury, keep away from, or deny the hurt or the fact of what has befell, it only gets greater difficult.

So many of us prefer to maintain our lives notwithstanding our pain. We conceal it and our scars with the aid of numbing materials like alcoholism, workaholism, overeating, and other strategies. Grief journeys are as person as the individual that undertakes them. The choice for self-care is part of grief that every one those who experience it percentage.

Grief can be felt in lots of approaches, together with physiologically, intellectually, spiritually, and psychologically. Grief can motive our bodies and mind to react in ways that encompass exhaustion, disturbed sleep, shifts in appetite and temper, memory, a loss of attention, and even hopelessness. Although dealing with this huge variety of feasible reactions may additionally seem daunting, several techniques may be applied to manipulate grieving reactions and keep on with every day life.

Emotions are what they're; they're infrequently right or terrible. Among the numerous emotions that might floor, isolation, disappointment, anxiety, perplexity, and wrath are all perfectly natural. Early in loss, emotions are often uncooked, however it is critical to allow them to be expressed. Attempting to suppress feelings frequently results in them later bursting in tons less most advantageous situations.

Grieving is a very non-public procedure. Accept that there is no set time table or magic recipe. It will take but lengthy it wishes to. Consider the compassion you would show a pal experiencing the equal loss, and expand your self the same forgiveness. It is tons better to go away room for a few flexibility in a single's commitments right now rather than taking up more obligations than is affordable.

Amid grief, it may be pretty smooth to forget about about one's personal physical needs. However, it is a important time to prioritize taking care of oneself. Even even though it can seem difficult, putting forth the effort to get sufficient sleep, consume nutritious ingredients, in shape in physical pastime, and deliberately loosen up can work miracles. Consider it like this: by means of retaining a wholesome

45

dependancy, you're making ready and preparing your self to address the new demanding situations you'll come upon all through it slow of grieving. Along with those measures, we usually recommend getting checked up. Tell your physician which you have just misplaced a cherished one.

Recognize that grieving is tough; it takes a lot of effort and may be draining. Even while we price ego extraordinarily (particularly in this region of the u . S . A .), it's far vital not to be afraid to ask for or obtain aid from the ones near you. Others had been worried and in reality want to help, but they are frequently unsure how or what to offer. Knowing somebody to open up to is especially critical due to the fact telling your tale out loud is important for restoration. Additionally, keep in mind that expert recommendation is also handy.

four.1 Relaxation Exercises May Help

Our frame's tissues and minds' fibers come to be entangled with the hurt, which reasons them to constrict and transform the ache into distress. The refusal to deal with our struggling with compassion or maybe forgiveness makes us unhappier and causes our lives to be out of music.

When you mourn the lack of a cherished one, your coronary heart isn't always the most effective organ affected. Most folks experience a physical collapse due to the frigid pain of loss. Although you may surely undergo the bodily results of grieving in your manner, a few standard responses encompass exhaustion, vomiting, shortness of breath, and compression within the chest and neck.

The body, regularly left out, can either be a supply of distress or a method of locating solace. Like a young toddler, the body will act out and make subjects worse if unnoticed. The chilly tightness for your joints and emotions can soften if you deal with your body with love and kindness. This will relieve physical ache while imparting a peaceful area on your mind. A chance to break out the worry and rumination that often accompany grief.

For maximum people, grief is arguably the maximum excessive shape of stress. We all understand the terrible consequences stress can also have on our bodies. The truth that our muscular tissues are demanding indicates that our frame is getting ready for combat, yet the handiest element we need to cope with is our worry! Thankfully, the pressure reaction may be stopped. The body can halt the fight-flight-freeze reaction to pressure when entreated to relax, and it could additionally undo the negative physiological results of strain.

Of course, unwinding will not regulate the truth which you lost. However, it can lessen your bodily discomfort whilst also relieving you of pressure. Try the workout listed under in a quiet, heat surroundings with out interruptions. You will practice this even as curled up on a mat or other floor coverings.

To stay heat, wrap your self in any other comforter. If it feels appropriate, positioned a pillow or wrapped blanket beneath your knees to ease the pressure on your decrease again.

Many people partner relaxation with vegging out in the front of the Television on the couch after a traumatic day. However, it does now not do a lot to lessen the bad influences of pressure. Instead, you have to cause your body's herbal calming reaction, a deep sleep-like condition that reduces stress, lowers your coronary heart fee and respiration charge, reduces your high blood pressure, and restores concord on your frame and thoughts. You can gain this by way of carrying out rest physical activities like yoga, tai chi, deep breathing, contemplation, and repetitive movement.

While you may determine to invest in a consultant rubdown, for example, most rest exercises may be carried out for my part or with the help of a cheap cellphone app or a unfastened audio down load. But it's miles vital to do not forget that no longer all of us responds well to a specific rest approach. We are all unique. The method that appeals to you suits your way of life and will let you concentrate so that you revel in rest is the best one. That means that locating the technique that works a good deal better for you can want trial and mistakes. Once you have got performed it, regular practice can assist decrease strain and tension, beautify sleep, growth energy and temper, and beautify your general health and health.

Relaxation Techniques

• Deep Breathing

Deep breathing, which emphasizes taking lengthy, purifying breaths, is a honest however effective relaxing approach. It is simple to examine, may be practiced practically everywhere, and gives an powerful method of lowering strain. Deep breathing is the idea of many different sorts of relaxation, which can be supplemented with different calming strategies like aromatherapy and song. While you may follow along side packages and audio downloads, you best need a few moments and a quiet area to loosen up or stretch out.

• Progressively Relaxing the Muscles

A -step innovative muscle relaxation method includes sequentially tensing and enjoyable diverse bodily muscle tissues. Regular exercise permits you to know intimately how one-of-a-kind sections of your frame sense under pressure and when they're completely relaxed. This would possibly assist you in responding to the primary indications of strain-related physical anxiety. Additionally, your mind will unwind as your frame does.

Breathing and revolutionary muscular relaxing can be used together to reduce anxiety in addition.

- Meditational Body Scan

This kind of meditation directs your awareness to numerous regions of your body. You start at your ft and start operating your manner up, just like sluggish muscle relaxation. You really deal with how every thing of your body feels without categorizing the sensations as "true" or "bad" in place of tensing and relaxing your muscle tissues.

- Visualization

In visualization, also known as intellectual meditation, you imagine a non violent putting in which you're free to allow cross of any tension and anxiety. This is a version of traditional meditation. Pick a vicinity that makes you sense relaxed, whether it's far a tropical lodge, an area you loved as a teen, or a peaceful forested glen.

You can use an app or audio record to help you together with your visualization sports, or you may practice on your very own. You also can decide to execute your visualization in complete silence or use listening to aids, inclusive of calming tune, a legitimate machine, or a report corresponding to your preferred location, which includes the wave sounds on a beach.

• Self-Massage

You are surely well privy to the great blessings of a skilled spa or gymnasium treatment on lowering pressure, easing ache, and easing muscular anxiety. With self-massaging or replacing massages with cherished ones, you can gain among the identical benefits at domestic or the office.

Try giving your self a quick massaging at your table among jobs, on the couch after a protracted day, or in sleep that will help you loosen up earlier than night time. You can use scented lotion or aromatic oils to result in rest or mix self-speak with meditation or deep rest techniques.

•

• Consciousness Training

In latest years, meditation has won giant recognition, receiving press insurance and endorsement from entertainers, corporate titans, and psychiatrists alike. And what precisely is mindfulness? By changing your awareness to what's occurring right now, mindfulness permits you to be absolutely present within the situation in place of stressing about tomorrow or obsessing approximately the past.

Mindfulness-based totally meditations were used for a long term to reduce strain, anxiety, despair, and other bad feelings. Some strategies help you turn out to be greater present via directing your attention to a unmarried, repeated pastime, inclusive of your breath or a few repeated terms. Some mindfulness practices urge you to cognizance and allow go of inner thoughts or sensations. Exercise, consuming, and other behaviors can all gain from practicing mindfulness.

It can also appear easy to practice mindfulness to maintain your interest inside the gift, however it takes attempt to benefit from it fully. When you begin to exercise, you'll probable be aware that your mind frequently go back for your issues or regrets. Do not give up, although. You are developing a brand new cognitive habit that could useful resource you in letting go of annoying approximately the preceding or the destiny every time you deliver your interest to the existing moment. When you first start out, using an software or audio record also can help you in concentrating.

four.2 Taking Care of Your Health & Diet

As you manipulate the strain of grief, a wholesome weight-reduction plan is important. That entails consuming many end result, greens, unprocessed foods, water, and other healthful beverages. Try eating greater frequently and in smaller portions if your desire is lacking. Any dietary gaps can be filled with a each day multivitamin.

Eating and grief cross hand in hand. Some people might also start eating less and lose their appetite. Other humans are extra inclined to bask in comfort eating, consuming extra than common. These reactions are pretty regular. However, you may start feeling out of control and that your consuming patterns negatively effect your physical and psychological disorders.

We study the relationship among food and grief beneath. We examine the capacity causes of your changing eating patterns and the options to be had to you should making a decision to accomplish that. You can also locate your self eating much less regularly if you lately lost any individual. Grieving regularly causes human beings to shed pounds.

According to studies, grieving might make you lose your starvation. You might discover which you do no longer need to eat, making it a nuisance. You would possibly notice which you come to be uninterested in beyond pastimes whilst suffering. Meals may additionally fall underneath this.

You frequently sense bodily and psychologically fatigued whilst going via grief. Finding the inducement to finish even the smallest activities may be pretty difficult. It is probably overwhelming to devise a meal, save for the products, put together, or maybe order takeaway.

It is hard to concentrate at the same time as you're experiencing intellectual suffering. Your grief will probable preserve you from eating as it will be in your mind an excessive amount of. This is specifically true in case you plan the burial and handle your loved one one's affairs. There can be a lot for your mind which you forget to consume.

When you're mourning, it's miles very natural to lose your hunger and devour less, however this could reason you to sense a whole lot worse. Even though it can seem difficult, taking care of yourself is vital while matters are tough. Food gives us with strength and helps healthy mind characteristic. Our intellectual health might also go through if we cross prolonged stretches with out food or consume insufficiently. Read those guidelines for handling a loss of appetite throughout a time of loss:

Create regular reminders for your smartphone to help you in recalling to make cereal, lunch, and dinner in case you discover which you are failing to accomplish that.

• Establish A Daily Schedule

You will not have to plan your food, which requires a intellectual attempt which you might not have in case you set up a schedule in which you eat at set up times for the duration of the day. You will increase the addiction of eating on that timetable if you persist with the agenda and no longer your feelings.

• Ask for Assistance

There will undoubtedly be a person looking to help you with the aid of cooking a few domestic-cooked meals due to the fact times of misery carry out the high-quality in human beings. Because you can store batch-cooked dishes like lasagna and chili in your fridge and freezer for some time, they are first-rate.

• Using Comfort Food to Deal with Loss

When mourning, some people flip to food for solace and devour greater than they generally might. Again, experiencing grief while overeating is very herbal. If you experience eating and discover it a source of pleasure, it seems that you would overeat and placed on weight whilst you are mourning.

• Consumption Generates Dopamine

Dopamine is one of the materials made within the brain that permits us to experience satisfied. It is scientifically proved to make us happier due to the fact eating reasons the mind to launch dopamine. Food consumption can momentarily reduce your suffering and enhance your mood whilst going through a horrible time after a cherished one.

• You Connect Comfort with Food

You might equate ingesting with feeling comforted and soothed if you have always trusted meals for solace. It isn't always surprising that you lodge to meals that will help you feel higher via one of the toughest times of your lifestyles—bereavement.

• Food Is Conveniently Available

You can be using a first-rate deal of time on the house, where a large quantity of food is available when you have these days experienced a loss. Your friends and circle of relatives can also have made damn positive you've got plenty of meals, which may also purpose you to consume extra than everyday.

four.Three Be Closer to Nature

After the loss of a close one, grieving is a normal technique. There are many extraordinary approaches to cope with your grief and the related feelings. Experts say that going outside is one of the first-rate coping techniques.

The physiological effects of natural sunlight hours and flora are concept to lessen heart rate and the stress hormone cortisol. Outside physical interest "permits for an boom in fantastic brain chemicals which includes dopamine, adrenaline, and endorphins due to the useful impact of the solar at the body's brain chemistry.

While accomplishing out of doors activities does not update getting professional assist for treating sadness encountered in the course of a loss, it allows guide neurochemical equilibrium and gives optimistic channels for the mourning method. There is a satisfying out of doors event for each person, whether you are generally active or stay a extra sedentary life.

Establish a Memorial Garden

One wonderful hobby to decorate bodily health is gardening. People will certainly receive more sunlight publicity at the same time as planting, which increases diet D intake and raises calcium, which is right for the immune system. Particularly whilst you plant a remembrance lawn, you may take advantage of gardening's health benefits whilst additionally honoring a deceased loved one. The best function is which you aren't required to do it by myself. By taking care of your memorial garden, you may spend time with the ones mourning the loss of a cherished one and maintain a connection to the outdoors.

Plant the flora, fruits, or veggies that your deceased cherished one preferred to create a place for introspection and remembrance on your memorial garden.

Exercise

Exercise is essential for enhancing general fitness, however it has additionally historically been related to raising mood, decreasing pressure tiers, and decreased stress, all of which promote stepped forward focus and sleep.

Many intellectual fitness practitioners advocate workout at some stage in tough times as it directly links to pressure discount.

The extra blessings of daylight and clean air come from workout out of doors. Yoga, trekking, riding, and taking walks are a few commonplace out of doors exercise pastimes which might be best for humans of all bodily abilities. Planning a brand new journey would possibly from time to time be an excellent manner to distract yourself from your loss.

Travel

Try a journey to a close-by nature hold for an extremely low-stress adventure. Take within the grandeur of the new scenery alone or with the employer while playing a simple picnic of your preferred dishes or the favorites of your deceased cherished ones.

Going to a brand new vicinity might also be proper for your health. The U.S. Travel Organization determined in a observe that journey complements one's view on life and mood. The effects display that 86 percent of travelers are content with their lives, compared to only 75 percentage of non-travelers.

Traveling's temper-improving benefits can useful resource people in overcoming strain and grief. Even apparently little reports, like driving your motorbike in a logo-new forest preserve or taking the correct photo of a well-known monument in a brand new region, can positively affect your mourning manner. While it is ordinary and sizable to mourn and grieve the loss of a cherished one, it is extraordinarily relevant to pursue happiness yet again actively.

According to a Stanford-led take a look at, human beings who have walked in herbal settings (as opposed to city ones) displayed a fairly lower degree of activity within the vicinity of the mind associated with depression. An individual is much more likely to sense depressed each time there's high electricity electromagnetic on this region; hence a decline in interest is useful. Studies have located a connection between introducing human beings to nature and quicker recovery instances, lessened stress, and relieved signs and symptoms of physical and mental illnesses. Even just looking at nature has health advantages.

Time away for reflection and processing is vital but tough to discover for most folks who're mourning. These sports provide us with the time and isolation required to technique our mind, whether or not taking walks or hiking a mountain. We can take gain of the peace with out being removed from the outdoor international. In addition, we can communicate aloud while vital, either to a loved one or to ourselves.

Sometimes, especially whilst we are dealing with grieving sentiments, we only want time to disengage from the sector that is getting increasingly more traumatic and bad. It can be hard for some human beings to unplug completely, but doing so is beneficial and healthful. We have the threat to enjoy the world with out such interruptions and misunderstandings while we take some time to understand the surroundings.

It may be hard to pin down just what it's miles in nature that promotes higher mental fitness. For one person, it could be the risk to procedure their emotions and thoughts at some stage in their by myself time. Another will respect the wreck from the town's busy pace and the resulting tension reduction. Another opportunity is that all it takes to break the vicious cycle of sadness and help someone re-hook up with oneself in a extra optimistic light is the sheer magnificence of lovely natural beauty.

And due to the fact sorrow is a non-public experience, there is no right or incorrect manner for a person to handle it. Moreover, spending time with nature may be incredibly pleasurable and beneficial for overcoming loss. Additionally, it really works nicely in assisting children in processing their sadness.

Four Follow a Set Routine

We begin looking after ourselves day by day with little effort on every occasion we feel nice. But while we go through a big loss, some things we typically take with no consideration, which includes our capability to care for ourselves, come to be a whole lot more challenging. Grieving people frequently suffer changes in appetite, sleep sample, electricity stage, recognition, and ability to attend to their frame. The grief method consists of it. The effects on these items might not always be the same because each tragedy is specific. What ought to you do if meeting those requirements is clearly tough for you? Try the under-listed dependent schedule. You is probably capable of comply with this ordinary on your own or require the assist of a friend you could name for guide. Always recollect to ask for assist in case you need it.

Get a bit of a blank sheet of paper and make a agenda. Your report have to consist of seven columns. Write the dates of the month above every row, beginning with Mondays. Beginning with the hour, you regularly rise up, and completing with the hour, you typically visit mattress and split each row into rows. Describe your standard day within the chart. Begin with the fundamentals:

- Your wake-up and bedtimes

- Travel time to and from paintings

- Job hours

- Regular food

- Domestic duties and interests

Try to include other things now, including time for grieving, workout, pursuits, and social interactions with friends and loved ones. So what does "time to grieve" truely imply?

If we can take out some time to cognizance on it, grieving is easier to manipulate. This does now not imply depicting which you ought to or can't enjoy any sorrow feelings earlier than your deliberate time. It implies that you attempt to concentrate your cognizance on what's in front of you while it isn't always your "grieving time." When you're to your "grieving moment," you can reflect to your loss and take steps in the direction of restoration. Keeping a magazine, chatting to a pal, touring a counselor, attending a grief aid community, talking with a pastor, surfing pictures, paying attention to music, and so on., are a few examples of "grieving time" hobbies. Now is the instant to nicely join and technique your feelings over your loss.

Ensure your timetable is as well-balanced with various sports as it will be as soon as you end it. To address your loss, you do no longer need to, for instance, turn into a party animal or a workaholic. Try to manipulate your timetable to allow for time for work, socializing with own family and buddies, snoozing, interests, and grieving. Keep as near this timetable as you could. When navigating the complicated variety of grief's emotions, adhering to a clean, measurable shape might be useful. To help you persist with your plan, do now not neglect to check in with a friend as important. Even with your greatest efforts, there may additionally from time to time be an imbalance. For instance, you would possibly sleep excessively or decide no longer to socialize as frequently as you meant to. This is a regular step within the procedure. The intention is to reap equilibrium so your sorrow does no longer begin to rule you.

Let's communicate a little bit approximately the essential components of self-care, specifically consuming, resting, and exercising. You want the strength to grieve, so consuming often and getting sufficient sleep are vital. It is additionally important to take some time to training session. Your system can go out of balance because of poor vitamins and poor sleep, that could purpose adjustments in mood and negative bodily potential. Exercise is crucial because it keeps your bodily health wholesome. Eating behavior may alternate when we're mourning, starting from excess to restricting calories.

If your tendency to overeat, strive to adhere to your meal timings as carefully as possible can and make most of your meals purchases from wholesome sources. Stick as carefully as possible for your mealtimes in case you generally tend to underneath-devour. Maintain simplicity in desire of food. The aim is to devour as a great deal nutritious meals as you may. If you and your household have to consume frozen food, order pizza, or enlist the help of a relative to prepare food, then that is what you ought to do. Recall that this is only brief.

You may not experience the urge or need to exercising similarly to ingesting. Fitness may be a splendid technique for some humans to address loss. Others find it hard. Spending plenty of time on the health club isn't notably essential. Regularly taking a short, 10-minute stroll may be pretty useful.

Sleeping patterns can variety from deep sleep to mild slumber. If you have got trouble falling asleep, try to permit yourself as a minimum thirty minutes to unwind before mattress. Cut the TV off. Give your self a moment to rest and simply breathe. Some individuals may additionally advantage from a bathtub before bed. Reading may also be useful to you. Try to set up a constant sample in which you go to mattress and awaken at the precise instances if you have a tendency to oversleep.

Keep in thoughts that grieving takes attempt. Although it could appear easy to put into effect those thoughts, it's far often not. To get via this procedure segment, try to offer your self a few shape. Anything isn't critical to execute it completely or effectively. Remember that this is simplest transitory and is your thoughts and psyche's reaction to and way of handling a loss. A therapist is often a completely useful teacher and source of help if you suffer with this process step.

Chapter 5: Tackling Loss Grief Trauma

Tackling loss trauma has never been less difficult as experts now increase the only recommendations and strategies. The first-class issue is that a touch self-assist can take care of maximum of your problems as far as such a type of trauma is worried.

five.1 Prefer Good Company

The toughest reviews in life are often the deaths of these we love and the pain they reason. Both one's intellectual and bodily fitness may also go through as a end result. Unfortunately, most groups call for that employees document lower back to work earlier than they're prepared to resume their "regular" exercises.

Experiencing loss whilst operating can be tough. Look at a few hints to help you in managing dropping a expensive one in case you find yourself in that situation. Even even though it has probably been impossible in an effort to stop thinking over your loved ones, you must not anticipate everyone on the office to be aware about your grief as soon as you return to work.

The truth is that, whether loss concerns a worker or a loved one of a worker, most organizations and businesses control the finality of life just as clumsily and badly as maximum people do. Because speaking approximately loss of life makes humans uncomfortable and often leaves us speechless, we regularly use slang phrases that deny it, say the incorrect aspect, or (worst nevertheless) say not anything.

Hence, it might be wrong to take into account that your business enterprise informed each person you have interaction with at paintings approximately dropping a loved one even as you were away. While a few groups might also inform all of the staff straight away, many others will inform your colleagues on your department or department or your direct boss and assume that news will "get about" earlier than you come to work.

One advantage of doing this in man or woman is that you could ask your coworkers to aid you whilst you are grieving. For example, you might inform humans that it is ideal to mention the call of your departed loved one round you, to pay respects, or to share their great reminiscences in the event that they pick out.

Grief remedy goals to guide the individual in shifting past their loss through helping them in grieving healthily, understanding and dealing with their emotions, and ultimately finding closure. The distinction between counseling and psychotherapy is commonly just a rely of semantics.

Discussions among the patient and the psychotherapist are utilized in counseling and psychotherapy to assist the customer in confronting psychological, intellectual, or behavioral demanding situations and finding solutions. However, "counseling" and "therapy" are sometimes hired in slightly unique contexts. Counseling is widely used to explain workshops where customers address greater difficult, pervasive, and persistent troubles, consisting of depressive episodes, tension, or addiction. Treatment is greater extensively used to refer to conversations where people cope with these troubles.

Consequently, despite the fact that grief remedy and counseling are basically the equal, "grieving therapy" is more likely to apply to meetings that clients participate in when they have issues with their grief which might be out of doors the standard variety of reactions.

For example, a widow may searching for grief counseling if she has issues adjusting to her husband's passing. Still, if she has ignored her urge for food and has trouble resting for weeks, it is probably a extra good sized issue for which she wishes grieving therapy.

While most persons grieving the lack of a pricey one do no longer need grief counseling, there are big potential advantages for folks that are hurting extra than normal. Grief counseling can assist someone in addressing their sturdy emotions and beginning the healing method if they had been distressed before the loss they skilled or if their sorrow is continual and impedes daily functioning.

Making sense of loss and coming to phrases with those emotions may be difficult. When you bear loss following a catastrophe or tragic incident, you frequently have a psychological and once in a while physical reaction known as grief. A type of professional remedy called grief counseling is supposed to help you in transferring thru the numerous stages and various emotions you can experience after a loss.

Many people eventually conquer or grasp grief. However, "complicated grieving" may additionally strike more or less 15% of those who lose a loved. You may additionally have signs and symptoms and signs of this form of sorrow for as much as one year or greater. The quantity of the signs and symptoms you may revel in varies depending at the instances of the loss and may differ from individual to character. It might be hard to finish your everyday sports and function normally if your grieving is complex.

The first step involves constructing trust with the man or woman to provide a steady and welcoming atmosphere where the bereaved can freely speak the statistics in their loss. Along with listening carefully to the mourning person, the counselor's second degree comprises probing detailed inquiries regarding the customer's reference to the deceased. Counseling could call for a distinctive approach if the healer and the deceased had a strained dating in preference to when there was an awesome rapport among them.

Not handiest adults who're handling loss benefit from grief counseling. Counselors who focus on grief work with humans who've lost a coworker, kids who're coping with the demise of a figure, buddy, or pet, hospice patients, couples or women who're grieving a miscarriage, and others who've skilled trauma.

Counseling Techniques for Grief

The grief counselor may additionally start the use of positive grief counseling procedures after the exact instances of the loss have certainly been satisfactorily decided, which can also include the following:

• Mentioning the Deceased Person

Grieving humans may also need a stable area to speak about their grief but cannot find one. A grief counselor should urge the bereaved to speak about the deceased's existence, including what it was like, who they cherished and cherished them, and their hobbies. What particular trends made them so specific (or even what makes them tough)?

• Separating Trauma from Grief

A grief counselor will assist a person experiencing trauma because of a memory or the statistics surrounding losing a beloved one in readjusting their angle on those memories and reframing their courting with the deceased to promote healthier mourning.

• Handling Guilt Feelings

Many human beings revel in remorse over their movements or inactions while a cherished one is around. To don't forget their cherished ones, a mourning person must be encouraged by using a grief counselor to surrender the shame or allow themselves forget about approximately them for a brief even as.

6.2 Acceptance and Commitment Therapy

Loss is part of lifestyles for all people. People sometimes go through a loss because of expected life transitions, but in other times, they may be recognised to engage in an unforeseen loss that could make them feel devasted and by myself. People searching for grief counseling may additionally have experienced various losses, including dying, marriage, job loss, or the loss of their baby because of a prison split. Others may are trying to find counseling because of transitory losses like leaving home, beginning a brand new activity, or having serious doubts about the cause of their life decisions.

In addition to disclosing losses associated with lifestyle, objectives, and aspirations, a person in search of counseling for despair is possibly to accomplish that. While the loss's diploma, intensity, and shape may additionally range, dealing with sorrow may also consist of letting move of once-carefully held hopes and goals. People regularly negotiate how their futures and goals may additionally materialize dramatically as they go through emotional pain.

Grief is a key a part of therapy exercise due to the fact people enjoy various existence losses, together with the passing of cherished ones, marriage, substance abuse, sickness, trauma, employment transitions, and regular life cycle changes. Most counselors will offer a few type of grief therapy in some unspecified time in the future in their careers. As they begin to lose their loved ones, the present toddler boomer generation is in all likelihood to want greater bereavement counseling. There may be a big demand for grief counseling offerings, raising the need for green grief counseling strategies and precious suggestions.

Acceptance and therapeutic intervention are one such paradigm and set of strategies that could deliver people gear to manage their grieving process. The time period "recognition and commitment remedy" (ACT) refers to a massive organization of broadly employed empirical evidence techniques and is a part of the "third wave" of conduct remedy. Spiritually, the ACT emphasizes that pain is important for the human experience and attracts suggestion from Eastern and Western religious traditions. Grief is a effective emotional nation rooted in communication, intimate communications, and a terrible occasion.

To realise and navigate their sorrow and consequently aid inside the procedure of recuperation, ACT might also provide counselors and customers strategies. ACT has been used with grieving humans to assist those going through complex, protracted sorrow practice mindfulness and embrace their stories. ACT aids grieving people in processing their thoughts as thoughts in preference to tendencies that outline them. Many bereaved human beings understand their ideas as reality. People who have experienced a intense loss can also sense their complete world has crumbled. They can discover it difficult to understand their component in this occasion. In assessment to the fake identification that sorrow produces, the ACT concept of the concept of self permits individuals to discover with and go beyond the experience of self and understand its more significance of their truth.

Individuals grieve their adjustments and grief in various methods on the grounds that there are various varieties of loss. Therapy affords clients with a secure region to grieve the loss and a platform to specific their struggling, hopes, and feel-making strategies. Numerous models can be used to direct grieving work. ACT is an emerging strategy that mixes theories from the fields of cognition and behavior in addition to meditation. The ACT paradigm handling mourning customers includes six middle levels. While supporting clients to empathize with and recognize the fact in their losses, this model gives a machine thru which counselors can gauge their cognizance and presence with people.

An essential therapy purpose is to find ideas that help patients in naming their grief and shifting toward healing due to the fact pain denial can worsen peoples' accidents in the course of instances of loss. In this manner, ACT can assist in making experience in their losses with the aid of honoring their reviews, expressing their feelings, and considering sparkling perspectives. People can inspire concordance amongst their values and upcoming recuperation steps by means of the usage of ACT.

6.3 Cognitive Behavioral Therapy

If your strain and grief are so deep that it interferes along with your capability to go about your normal activities, or if it does not get better with time, you might need to talk to a consultant.

Interventions from cognitive behavior remedy (CBT) can be applied to help humans in managing easy or complex grieving. People would get hold of commands on slowly returning to their normal habits. Gradual publicity to events they may have prevented because of the frightening recollections is a key element of CBT for complex grieving.

Continuous avoidance maintains effective feelings in check, whereas touch with those occasions gradually causes emotions' electricity to vanish. It has been validated that cognitive behavioral remedy, which uses exposure and cognitive therapy to combat avoidance, is extra green than assisting counseling.

Evidence-primarily based research for PTSD and hard bereavement the usage of cognitive behavioral remedy (CBT) and the CBT-REBT technique for treating grief are reviewed. A CBT-REBT-based totally intervention aims to sell a healthful adjustment to loss after death. There is a differentiation among healthful (adaptive) and unhealthy (irrational) bereavement procedures.

The enduring bonds perspective emphasizes loss and grieving as a lifelong technique of growth that serves to preserve a continuing dating with the dead. Furthermore, the later methods emphasize that there's nobody predictable course thru the grieving and view it as an character experience as opposed to looking ahead to a predefined course and cease of loss. Similar to this, the "legendary" 12-month length in the course of which people are purported to resume "regular existence" has changed, and what is currently common as regular "grief paintings" is a much longer and greater worried manner.

As a result, grieving for the individual that has handed away and developing a brand new sense of purpose for lifestyles without them are both common components of the private grief system. The intensity of disappointment that doesn't bring about the absorption of the loss but rather in recurrent stereotypical conduct and reduced functioning is known as grieving. Traumatic activities surrounding the loss of life are one chance aspect for complex mourning, and those situations can also result in special feelings like melancholy, stress, and PTSD.

These frequently coexist and overlap, highlighting the importance of assessment earlier than beginning therapy. Research has paved the way for setting apart intense grieving from depression, which incorporates obsessive considering the deceased, crying, non-stop yearning, and looking for the lacking man or woman. The implications of this take a look at encourage the usage of opportunity remedy methods for despair and grieving, along with therapy with a caring and supportive cognizance.

Chapter 6: Therapies For Grief Loss

Trauma

Each man or woman's revel in with mourning is specific, and it can be challenging to inform when everyday grief becomes complex grief. How long earlier than extreme grieving may be diagnosed is a subject that mental health professionals are currently operating on.

When the depth of your grieving has not subsided inside the months that accompanied the demise of a loved one, you'll be experiencing stressful strain. Some mental health vendors become aware of complicated grief whilst sorrow is powerful, prolonged, and incapacitating after a year.

Complicated grief and most important depression proportion many characteristics but can range extensively. Depression and hard grief can on occasion coexist. A thorough mental and physical examination is frequently executed considering that figuring out the right prognosis is essential for receiving the proper treatment.

Grief counseling or therapy is the primary method of treating grief. These phrases would possibly check with numerous treatments, despite the fact that they may be synonymous. While remedy more often refers to the shipping of therapy (communicate remedy) by a specific remedy modality, counseling is a widespread concept that can also apply to recommendation-giving and religious support.

Any counseling or remedy can provide a person experiencing regular sorrow the understanding, aid, and direction they need to get via the grief procedure. Plans for treating grief often assign various tasks to diverse tiers. Working via denial, letting cross of guilt or blaming, digesting emotions, and handling secondary losses are a few examples of these sports.

A therapist generally needs specialized education in psychotherapy strategies to correctly deal with tough sorrow. Trauma, accrued grief, or different variables that can lead to protracted or persistent grieving reactions may be the concern of remedy for grief. Recent research monitor that the previously believed linear and everyday stages of mourning are not usually present. The idea that mourning is a way of rediscovering reason after a loss is still widely recognized.

When deep emotions of sadness, isolation, dread, fear, guilt, wrath, anger, and disgrace stay unresolved, psychology characterizes grieving as complex. Acute sorrow is the introductory segment of loss that controls life, and such lengthy periods of acute grieving hinder the ability to orient and create new which means. The enjoy renders it not possible for the bereaved to check a lifestyles with out their cherished one; everything else appears nugatory, and other people are left feeling disillusioned and powerless.

More than uncomfortable silences or platitudes are wanted while a person is going through this type of lengthy and profound mourning; they want "connection, for talking and tale accumulating." They recognize what has passed off but can not be given it, and they could regard mourning as a burden rather than everyday human emotion. Even the maximum experienced physicians find the relationship between disappointment and mourning complex and frequently complicated. As a result, receiving a mental fitness prognosis within the first two months after losing a cherished one is frequently prevented.

There are distinctions as well. The grieving man or woman's subject with ideas, photographs, and recollections of the deceased is a commonplace way to recognize grief. However, someone with intense depressive disease has a tendency to be obsessed on poor self-communicate, depressing thoughts, and a feel of worthlessness.

Support and Coping

Even whilst it is vital to have proper help for excessive sorrow, these coping mechanisms can also be useful to you:

Adhere on your treatment time table

Attend treatment periods on time, and use the abilities you've got discovered. Take capsules as prescribed, if important. Use and learn pressure control techniques. Depression, binge consuming, and different dangerous mind and behaviors can result from chronic stress.

Ensure Your Well-Being

Get enough sleep, have a balanced weight loss program, and unwind. Do normal exercising. Stress, melancholy, and fear can all be reduced via power schooling. Do no longer are searching for solace in drink or tablets.

Speak with Your Religious Community

Adhering to religious customs or practices, rituals, or spiritual leader steering may additionally carry you solace.

Socialize

Keep in contact with the individuals you want to be with. They can offer consolation, a sofa to cry on, or some shared laugh to lift your spirits.

Prioritize Important Events or Anniversaries

The passing of a loved one may convey up unpleasant reminiscences of vacations, anniversaries, and different special events. Find unique activities to consider, have fun, or honor the loved one that gives you solace and inspiration.

Obtain New Abilities

Try to analyze these activities for your personal if, for instance, you closely rely upon a cherished one to manage the price range or the cooking. As wanted, seek advice from circle of relatives, friends, or professionals. Find neighborhood resources and training as nicely.

Sign Up for A Support Network

After a loss, you may not be organized to enroll in a guide community right away, but as time passes, you would possibly find solace in different human beings's tales and develop deep connections.

Many people are uncertain of the way to guide a bereaved individual. They are puzzled to comfort the grieving and help them feel better. These nicely-intentioned moves could pass incorrect. People mourning can also by chance be harm or offended with the aid of saying, "At least they are in a higher position."

You aren't required to mention something to someone who wishes assistance handling disappointment. When a person is grieving, once in a while whilst the nicest factor you could do is just pay attention to them even as not making them feel right. People who are grieving regularly address powerful emotions that disappointed others. Others could subtly tell them they need to no longer sense as they do and ought to no longer maintain lower back on their grief presentations. Creating a safe surroundings for a person mourning to specific their emotions can be noticeably beneficial.

Such a version in addition clarifies a way to assist a loved one going through grief. This perspective indicates that human beings require assistance with greater than honestly the mental consequences of loss. People should learn how to deal with different losses once a cherished one passes away, such as changes to their character and financial state of affairs. These changes may sense daunting. Even routine tasks like cleansing and cooking can end up overwhelming whilst grief is robust. Helping with these tasks can appreciably improve someone's scenario.

6.5 Group Therapy

Some human beings may additionally are searching for counseling for the primary time after losing a cherished one; in the past, they will have treated other difficulties in life by using getting assistance from family individuals and different internal abilities.

However, the sadness and trouble of losing a liked one can be so wonderful that it exceeds our capability for self-sufficiency. After a major loss, there may be neither a wrong nor right way to grieve. In fact, numerous variables affect how we grieve, including our character, the kind of connection we had with our departed, and the situations surrounding their passing. The level of social aid, coping mechanisms, history of mental contamination, and cultural and spiritual historical past all impact the bereavement experience.

Group remedy contributors advantage understanding approximately the grief system and help one another in constructing bridges to the future. The satisfactory form of mourning is whilst it will become a shared social emotion. Participating in a set offers the threat to advantage aid networks from other grieving people who can recognize the hardships of loss. People who've misplaced an vital dating, together with a determine, sibling, partner, youngster, or different intimate friend or relative, gain from organization periods.

We need no longer provide self-assist sessions; all of our classes are facilitated through trained experts. Psychotherapy permits whiners to strive out one of a kind methods of referring to others in a safe putting. A therapist is also available to assist as required. Furthermore, group therapy allows you to advantage from others' reviews and recognize how individuals with unique worldviews and social dynamics have interaction.

Even even though experiencing sadness is a common human emotion, all people's grief is particular. You can better understand your loss and communicate the variety of emotions that accompany transition via institution therapy. Let psychotherapy help you in finding your equilibrium as you discover new ways to re-engage with existence. The institution is one of a kind because it specializes in healing aspects of grief rehabilitation and is run by way of a qualified therapist. As a end result, the revel in is going in addition than the tremendous, albeit short, effects of having social guide. Establishing a stable and steady healing surroundings falls on the group chief(s). To that goal, before the group start, we need to conduct a face-to-face interview with every applicant.

Group counseling is one remedy recommended assisting human beings going via complex sorrow. People grieving or who have misplaced a person frequently experience by myself because difficult grief reactions can negatively impact social help. Friends and circle of relatives regularly display subject for and assist to the mourning man or woman inside the aftermath of a loss. Nevertheless, the ones going through tough sorrow could put too much strain on their social networks for aid. Stress can doubtlessly isolate the suffering person and alienate their social circle. Grief peer help seems to be a appropriate substitute for conventional social networks.

Additionally, corporations may be an opportunity to learn coping mechanisms, strain-discount techniques, and a cathartic outlet. Grief businesses also are often quick, which may also provide some comfort to the struggling man or woman.

Counseling corporations for addressing traumatic strain frequently comply with certainly one of three major theoretical strands: psychoanalytic, relational, or cognitive-behavioral.

The interpersonal technique is every other properly-appreciated organization remedy fashion for coping with tough grief. The main desires of this model are to speed up the recovery procedure and aid the grieving person in regaining pursuits and connections. People are invited to mirror, speak the situations and outcomes of those occurrences, and look at their feelings and experiences about the loss. To recognize the modern-day relationship demanding situations, relationship patterns also are investigated. Similar to psychoanalytic group remedy, ambiguity toward the deceased is a key factor of the grieving technique in relational institution therapy. To encourage change, uncertainty desires to be mentioned and expressed.

Chapter 7: Rewiring Your Brain

One of the best strategies to handling loss trauma is to move for the movements that grow to be developing effective wondering styles for you. Rewiring your mind with positivity is the want of the hour in such conditions and may assure a hit remedy.

7.1 Set Your Goals

After suffering a excessive loss, intention-placing is simply as important as at any other factor in existence. People often describe a loss of enthusiasm as a grieving sign. During this era, setting up small, immediate desires can be important. Short-term targets may every so often be tiny steps taken in the direction of a larger goal. One might find optimism and things to sit up for by means of daydreaming approximately and making plans for long-time period goals. Think approximately setting up each a short-time period and long-term goal.

Realistic and conceivable dreams should be set. Discuss your targets with someone who will encourage and inspire you to perform them. To help you stay responsible, ask your customer service agent to check in with you as soon as every few months. When you reach out for a positive aim, set a new, more attainable one and relish the sense of fulfillment, no matter how modest. Whether you are going through a crisis to your lifestyles, grieving, or simply appreciating the street of lifestyles, aim making plans is critical in your fitness.

We advantage cause from our goals. Numerous goals must be met at the course to one's motive or restoration. Goals can give direction, specifically while existence turns into ambiguous.

Goals are the milestones on the street to success, whether or not you are attempting to get via crises someday at a time or have a massive plan for your life, home, business, or ministry.

Establishing goals and a timeline for each are required for a success purpose-setting. When your goals are vague, it's miles hard to photo them. Finding the power to behave is made extra challenging with the aid of this. Another signal of sadness is a lack of concept. We all experience loss in my opinion, which makes it difficult to overcome. The grief technique can be handled pretty differently from man or woman to person. Establishing practicable dreams permit you to get over your loss for this reason. By setting up affordable targets for oneself, you can pass at your pace while being held liable for feeling appropriate.

Setting SMART goals is one approach to navigate the grief manner. Even going to the supermarket might turn into a maze of recollections, reminiscences, tension assaults, and computations. Or, to place it every other way, you do now not just go to the nearby grocery store. It is extremely demanding because we will keep in mind what it became like earlier than things became so tough—earlier than carrying the burden of grief on the whole thing else.

We need to encompass disappointment while placing desires for lifestyles following a loss. Any dreams we make after a vast loss ought to take sadness into account due to the fact it's miles an inescapable thing of our lifestyles. This calls for us to rethink the whole of our pre-loss targets via the prism of loss and to create all the publish-loss dreams with grief integrated as a middle factor.

There are many things to don't forget, so take a moment to relax and give yourself space and time to make desires even as grieving.

Are you sure you need to reach this aim?

Undoubtedly, we have to finish sure responsibilities. We must contend with our food, garments, and housing needs. If we've got pets or kids, we ought to take care of them. We ought to take a sleep. Further than that, fantastically, extra pursuits than we count on are optional.

Before the loss, we should have evolved objectives due to the fact we notion we should. Others may additionally have looked on us to fulfill particular duties or roles. Even yet, we'd have made plans for ourselves to visit grad school or cross on holiday with out understanding how so much loss might have an effect on such sports. Ask yourself, "Is this objective some thing I absolutely want to do?" as you consider it. If the response is "No" or maybe "Not at the moment," be unhappy about it and toss it out, delegate it to someone else, or put it aside to think about later.

Play round with the idea of time.

After a loss, time should seem like an infinite tormentor, however do no longer be hesitant to entertain the notion that time may additionally be an best friend. Ask yourself, "Is it possible to alter the deadline in this?" in terms of your pursuits.

Think about the time you could permit yourselves to complete a assignment. Time might not be with you in case your goal has an expiration date, along with getting pregnant or hiking the Camino Santiago earlier than you lose your bodily ability. However, other targets, which include clearing your credit debt, finishing a race, or even buying food, will be behind schedule for numerous years. You can enjoy the time you'll have spent pursuing that goal to unwind and grieve your loss.

How may want to I make things a great deal less complicated, ask your self?

This isn't always the same as asking for "How can I scam" or "How can I have an effect on the system," to be clean. It is a reputation that grieving is difficult. Additionally, the person you are nowadays has special requirements and capacities than the man or woman you had been in the beyond.

Grief will on occasion triumph. There may be days whilst the ache will precede your objective, regardless of how crucial it's miles to you. So rather than anticipating disappointment to lurk within the background even as you try to flow forward, expect it to show up alongside the manner.

Can you're taking stock as soon as every week rather than each day, for instance? Can you spread out writing a thesis over six weeks in preference to in a 4-day, caffeine-fueled frenzy? Can you location an order for shipping or contact an keen neighbor who has been inquiring for help in preference to traveling to the supermarket yourself?

Give up, hoping that reaching this objective will carry you joy.

This is a widespread problem; you should consist of it to your aim-setting procedure following a loss. When sadness is present, the dopamine receives excessive that comes with completing tasks, getting a promotion, or figuring out your dreams can also feel insufficient or absent as compared to the life before the loss. The strain and surprise of grief would possibly dampen satisfaction and satisfaction, that is a herbal sensation.

You may reach your mission. Possibly no longer. Please recognize that it isn't your fault for no longer trying. Not because you lacked enough preference, even though. It is likewise no longer so because the objective you set up turned into unachievable or due to the fact you probably did not installed enough time or effort to achieve it. Even surviving lifestyles after loss is difficult, let alone placing and achieving dreams.

7.2 Own Your Responsibilities

It is probably difficult to recognize and assist a mourning friend, member of the family, or coworker. Because we might also fear mentioning the incorrect component or saying nothing, the grieving person can also feel alienated and alone.

If you haven't suffered the loss of a pricey one, you can have unreasonable expectations about the mourning character's emotions and how quickly they must resume their normal things or circulate on with their lives.

Despite the many things you can do or say to help a person, bear in mind that everybody's experience of sorrow is particular. Some of your ideas and hints might be proper, while others may not. Ask the individual mourning what they require or preference in case you are unclear a way to support them. Simply expressing your problem and choice to assist them may be pretty reassuring.

When aware about someone's misery, we clearly want to place matters proper for them. But the fact is that you cannot 'repair' someone else's unhappiness after a loved one passes away. There are items you could do to offer consolation and aid to a bereaved character at this attempting time, but there is not some thing you may say to help them sense better over their loss.

The maximum unique assistance you could offer is an open ear. Let the person who has misplaced a loved one talk and explicit their sadness as they need to. This should contain sobbing, yelling, giggling, expressing sorrow or regret, or taking part in pressure-relieving sports like planting or on foot.

Put all of your power into listening compassionately and attentively.

Allow humans to specific their disappointment in the approaches which might be maximum comfortable for them. Do now not criticize or disagree with their reactions to the loss of a cherished one. It is cruel to criticize how a person expresses their disappointment due to the fact that it'd discourage them from speakme to you approximately their feelings.

Do not press them to speak if they do no longer experience love it. Keep in mind which you provide comfort to them in reality by way of being there. Sitting quietly along is also beneficial.

Remember the significance of personal contact. It may be useful to maintain the guy's hand or hug them but ensure it is suitable to them first.

Balance is important for colourful, right fitness grieving. It will help if you stability the time spent seeking to paintings to your grief and the time you spend handling your daily responsibilities. You need to also stability the time you devote to others and your quiet time. You have to strike a balance among soliciting for help and worrying for your self. Concentrating on one companion in these pairs will cause a detour.

Look at a few thoughts that different humans have used to assist them grieve healthily. Pick those that work quality for you or devise a self-care regimen. Remember that mourning is an evolving system; it calls for energy, which you may possibly need to divert from your everyday activities momentarily. You must method yourself with the equal consideration, compassion, and love you will display a near friend in a comparable situation.

Although grieving can be excruciatingly painful, maximum humans (among 85% and ninety%) discover that they can finally cope with their loss with the assistance in their family, colleagues, and psychological capital and do now not require professional help.

However, there are times when the occasions surrounding the death might also had been extremely scary, together with a traumatic, surprising, or abrupt dying. In different cases, additional elements may additionally make the mourning specifically acute or tough. If your pal or member of the family appears to be having trouble managing their every day life through the years, you can suggest they are trying to find professional assistance.

7.Three Try Being More Social

Grief is a complex feeling that is complete of paradoxes.

While it seems like time is moving slowly, it isn't. We try to avoid demanding approximately dying despite the fact that we cannot help but reflect onconsideration on it. We are each strong and susceptible. We are susceptible even whilst we're sturdy.

Our assignment of mourning includes accepting and appreciating those crucial paradoxes, in addition to others. Equilibrium and returned-and-forth are key right here. While there's no accepted method suitable for all people, you'll discover that striving each day to find the equilibrium that works for you may help you flow forward.

Many people are familiar with grieving by myself. We regularly retreat inner whilst we're torn aside each spiritually and emotionally. Early grief creeps up on you like a fog. We can also regularly find ourselves in a while entangled in our inner sensations and mind. That is usual.

When grieving, we require quiet, on my own time to method our emotions and ideas. Sometimes we should pursue solitude to sluggish down and focus internal deliberately. It isn't a curse to be on my own, no matter what we could have been thinking. It is a privilege. We are by myself when we're born and alone while we bypass away. Each people is a special individual and a infant of the cosmos.

Grieving on my own is both critical and healing. Nevertheless, if you continuously divert yourself, hold busy, or come to be connected to different people to avoid being on my own, you could be getting rid of your herbal, important soreness. You is probably blockading out the silent, internal voice that tells you to gradual down, appearance inward, and pay extra interest to it. You may be ignoring your soul and spirit. Your grieving system will then stall. You emerge as mired in denial and evasion.

Always keep in thoughts that both too little and too much isolation may be adverse during a time of grief. The griever who totally closes off from the out of doors international and refuses to accept and acknowledge the help of others can likewise emerge as caught.

To accept and get hold of help from peers, loved ones, associates, and coworkers is certainly one of our fundamental desires at some point of a time of grieving. Thanks to their empathy, we may additionally convey our important and natural pain to others. We are shifting closer to recuperation whilst we discuss our sorrow and relate our love-and-loss experiences.

Humans require organisation; consequently, a assist community at some stage in a tough time is important. We are social beings, and our connections supply existence importance. Our grief bears witness to this truth. Our lives had reason due to the relationship we shared with the deceased. Other partnerships in our ongoing lifestyles are the identical way. We sense lonely while there aren't any pals. After dropping a special person, mainly one who have been part of our regular existence, isolation can be difficult. Being on my own hurts. We have to learn how to hook up with others to fight our loneliness.

We can create new habits for spending time with our buddies, own family, buddies, coworkers, colleagues, people from our neighborhood network, people who proportion our hobbies, and others. Concentration on connecting makes us experience less on my own and offers us hearing ears whilst we want to proportion our sorrow.

During our times of mourning, the effect of provider we want and obtain aids in creating a meaningful bridge that leads us into the future. Death may additionally have ended a unique connection, however we will still build and decorate new connections. While they could never fully update the deceased, those individuals can and will repair that means to our lifestyles.

7.Four Get Rid of Procrastination

There are advantages to residing in a technological age. But while we want to keep away from and do something we understand we need to be doing, it would provide the best diversion. We have instantaneous get admission to to statistics that is a consistent temptation for diversion. Having a lot availability these days makes it challenging to apprehend that now not all things essential can provide immediate gratification.

Procrastination is said to have persisted throughout the records of humankind, albeit the methods it manifested itself have evolved. It has been expected that greater than 20 percent of Americans are chronic procrastinators, making it the addiction of the Fifth of the humans in a country.

Procrastination generally occurs while a task seems impossible to finish and awakens our outstanding emotions. From apathy to melancholy to wrath to uncertainty to inadequacy—and the entirety in among—those irrational emotions may arise. When a person lacks the talents to deal with terrible emotions that may emerge, they may avoid the situation that delivered on the feelings, delaying finishing the undertaking. Anybody who knows they may enjoy these emotions will put off chores truely due to the fact they do now not have the way to deal with them. However, procrastinating can negatively impact our mental health whenever we eliminate chores that we recognise we must be doing because it makes us sense unprepared and careless.

Establish A To-Do List

Organizing oneself is one of the critical matters you can accomplish for yourself. Make lists, join in an organisation path, or get an organizer. Whatever fits you, do it. Keep it easy; this is my one piece of advice. Your organizational device might be but some other responsibility to avoid if it's far overly hard.

Do It Now

Get into a sporty attitude the next time you pay attention yourself thinking, "I can accomplish this later." Do it now! Do it now at the same time as overcoming your emotions. No amount of pleasure from delaying it'll examine to the thrill you may have while you finish.

Plan The Incentive Time

Your thoughts may additionally wander as you whole your obligations and consider the whole thing you'd opt to be doing. Knowing which you have set out time for rewarding sports will make it a great deal less difficult in an effort to awareness on your project.

Rethink Your Goals

Overcoming procrastinating may be hampered by using perfection and the perception that matters have to always be completed in a specific manner. In the very subsequent instance, you discover yourself using words like "need to" or "should," take into account if these constraints are ones you are putting yourself or whether or not they represent accurate depictions of the situation.

7.5 Make Nature Your Friend

An detail soothing about the surroundings makes our lives less disturbing. In a duration of loss, the perception of being a aspect of some thing bigger than oneself can be consoling. Nature soothes the soul and is incredible for assisting inside the restoration of loss. Outside existence ceremonies are desired because of their deeper importance and serene, beautiful environment.

Many people have observed therapy in nature, but what is the only method? Is it simply beautiful in terms of look? Or is there a non secular element similar to how water has therapeutic homes? There are numerous blessings to convalescing within the environment, from language to images. Even small quantities of time spent in nature all through the day might be beneficial for your fashionable nicely-being.

Studies have determined a connection among humans new to nature and less strain, quicker quotes of recovery, and alleviating signs and symptoms of medical and intellectual issues. Grieving humans regularly yearn to be outdoor and inside the barren region. It seems practical due to the fact grieving is not unique from different emotional states in which making an investment time outdoors is useful.

The cycle of existence is represented by way of nature. Roses, forests, plants, and gardens are examples of herbal additives that have long played a large function in our rituals associated with loss of life. There is an growing fashion toward shifting the funeral home surroundings out of doors because the calming sensation of merging with the environment allows with tension and melancholy.

Whenever you're along with your family or in your very own, breathe within the smooth air, sense the heat on your cheeks, and take within the world's beauty whilst remembering the one you love one with each step you are taking.

Grief can be felt in any way, no matter incorrect or proper. We all searching for significance and serenity in our unique approaches, however with the aid of going in touch with Mother Earth, you may flow past your emotions, experience at extra ease, and start grieving again.

7.6 Be More Optimistic in Life

Living with grief is difficult as every day passes; but, when a brand-new yr is beforehand of us, it can be even more hard. Your emotions of emptiness or loneliness after dropping a dear you'll make you hesitant to face the approaching year.

Grieving human beings could find it hard to take pleasure inside the holiday festivities as others start resolutions and seem to guide normal lives. Others can also worry approximately their ability to stand similarly obstacles, while some may be frightened of what the coming 12 months may additionally carry.

A tremendous technique permit you to get returned on path closer to embracing loss and coming across serenity, even though the beginning of the brand new 12 months might also suggest various matters to specific individuals. Grief drains the body and thoughts if the loss become foreseen or now not. It hurts when you lose a person, regardless of what degree of their existence your expensive one become at when they died away.

Be patient with yourself as you enter the brand new yr. When grieving, do no longer sense compelled to participate in sports or to share your emotions in case you are not ready. Try to loosen up your emotions via substituting affirmations for unfavorable thoughts. Even shortly after the loss, the ones who have experienced a loss experience a surprising quantity of fantastic emotions. In one studies on managing a newborn's demise, almost fifty percentage of the parents reported feeling happy 3 months following the loss of life.

Positive emotions do not need to be sturdy or final for a long term to have a high-quality effect. Mourners who revel in a huge amount of bad sentiment and only a small quantity of exceptional emotion fare higher than people who experience no tremendous emotion. Both fantastic and bad feelings can arise simultaneously and independently of one different. In controlling melancholy and other grief-associated horrific feelings, high quality emotions are crucial.

Individuals have a greater threat to revel in less unhappiness and suffering within the future if they show more satisfactory emotions in the initial few months after the loss. Focusing on satisfied feelings as opposed to painful ones offers mourners a intellectual ruin or reprieve and enables them to regain strength.

Positive emotions can help people deal with loss better. Mourners can better deal with and pass forward with the essential sports once you have some space from poor feelings and being healed and refilled by means of satisfied feelings. Positive feelings are extra challenging to sense after a few sorts of losses than others. For example, those who lose a cherished one all of sudden are more likely to feel negative feelings than people whose loved one died as anticipated. Even though experiencing unsightly matters is probably tough, you get more potent when you go on along with your existence without people, matters, or instances you used to have. You can develop the capability to address tough problems in the destiny with the aid of going thru a loss and trying to move on.

Not by using your self! There might be help networks available for your community to assist you in getting via any tragedies or losses you've got experienced. There are many forums where people come together to discuss their common reports on the net if you are not prepared to discuss things face-to-face or cannot locate the correct sort of support network. Tell us your story. To convince yourself that you can accomplish it too, inquire how others overcame tough situations.

Loss can occasionally supply way to sparkling opportunities. There is nothing incorrect with searching for methods to enhance or modify your life following a traumatic occasion, regardless of your initial emotions of guilt or selfishness. When a love engagement ends or a person you were caring for passes away; you may have more time to spend with colleagues or pursue pursuits you had been putting off. If a calamity has triggered you to lose your private home, you would possibly need to transport to the place of your ideal domestic.

It nearly appears herbal to concentrate at the grief you are experiencing because of losing someone you like. You can practice appreciation for those activities through reflecting at the satisfied instances you had with your pet or a person else. It may be even greater useful to have a pal or member of the family who is also grieving your loss accompany you in your recollections. Perhaps you two will be capable of snigger simultaneously.

After dealing with a horrible situation, treating yourself can help you in recalling how to sense higher and go back you to a function wherein you could experience all the pleasant deeds you offer. It does no longer be counted whether making a decision to do some thing exciting or peaceful; what subjects is that you are to do what you like.

You can assist keep a loved one's reminiscence by creating a tribute for his or her passing. You should determine to prepare a fundraising occasion of their honor, place a tree in certainly one of its favourite spots, dangle their photographs in your home, begin a memorial internet site or Facebook page, interact in some of their favorite hobbies, or even get a tattoo of them.

After a demanding occasion, it's far common to have issues adjusting to daily existence. Nevertheless, if weeks or months have surpassed and you still can't appear to perform or do not know a way to feel properly, it's far critical to get help.

Chapter 8: Never Leave Loss Grief

Unattended

One should by no means take grief with no consideration, as it may always have various influences in multiple ways. Your social and expert existence can be disturbed, and you will not be capable of carry out as according to your goals in lifestyles. Therefore, it must in no way be left unattended, and lengthy-time period solutions must be carried out.

3.1 Long-Term Impacts of Loss Grief

It isn't always a not unusual expertise that grief is a complete physical experience. But grieving can also have bodily results, just as it can effect intellectual health. Physical symptoms might not accompany some forms of grieving. However, profound grieving could have destructive effects which might also feel more physiological than anything else, which include those brought on with the aid of the loss of a child or a dating.

Various signs and symptoms of intellectual infection and troubles can be delivered on via grief. Sadness, loneliness, and fear can be among them. If you're struggling with sorrow or different associated emotions, speakme with a good therapist or counselor can be beneficial. Knowing the symptoms of grief to look out for might also assist you deal with any repercussions you could encounter and simplicity them.

1. Heart Issue

In many circumstances, extreme strain can result in heart problems. But grieving carries particular dangers for the coronary heart. According to one examine, losing a beloved one will increase a person's danger of a heart attack. This causes it to imitate the signs of a coronary heart assault, such as chest discomfort and shortness of breath, but it's far only transitory. Treatment is to be had for folks that suffer from damaged coronary heart syndrome. They may also determine to wait a few weeks for the situation to vanish.

Note which you have to see your health practitioner rule out greater severe causes if you have heart troubles or shortness of breath for an prolonged time. Any additional excessive or pervasive physical manifestations of grief are also valid.

2. Reduced Immunities

Some humans get the flu or the common cold when beneath excessive stress. During a time of intense mourning, they'll find out they may be extra at risk of the identical ailments. This is because disappointment can weaken the immune device in adulthood.

According to a 2014 study, grieving older individuals who had misplaced a partner, mainly, were not able to keep a healthy stability of strain hormones. They consequently have diminished neutrophil characteristic. This suggests that older men and women are less likely to create unique forms of white blood cells during the grief process, making them greater liable to infections.

three. Body Pain and Aches

Grief regularly manifests physically as pains and aches. Back pain, joint ache, migraines, and stiffness can all be delivered on by way of grief. The exuberant amount of strain chemical substances which are generated for the duration of the grief method is what causes the ache. The muscle tissues they come across are successfully greatly surprised by means of them. Similar to how coronary heart circumstance syndrome influences the body, stress hormones. Grief-related aches and pains need to subside over the years. Talk to your doctor in the event that they keep for a long time.

four. Digestion Problems

Stressful periods can hurt the digestive machine. It is simply too traditional to show to meals for solace at some point of worrying times or feel nauseous whilst concerned. These signs and symptoms, in conjunction with others, which include a loss of appetite, disordered ingesting, vomiting, and inflammatory bowel disease, are added on via grief.

Knowing that grief is responsible for those signs and symptoms can make them disappear. When you locate you haven't eaten all day due to your despair or feel the want to devour while you are disenchanted, it is able to be a sign which you need to agenda a go to with a certified mental fitness expert or a pal or relative.

5. Ill-Appropriate Coping Methods

One harmful coping method humans may want to use throughout mourning is ingesting or undereating. Some can also pose a more hazard than others. Individuals may additionally flip to materials like cigarettes or alcohol because excessive utilization could have bad long-term effects on the lungs and liver. Others would possibly use capsules, self-damage, or have interaction in other unstable behaviors. These coping strategies can probably seriously and completely harm the mind and frame. You should searching for out a close friend, member of the family, or educated professional for aid if you routinely have interaction in those sports to deal with your sorrow.

6. Sleep Issues and Tiredness

According to a 2017 look at, spouses who misplaced a loved one to suicide have been much more likely to revel in sleep troubles. The brain and frame are designed to relax and repair throughout sleep. It might be extraordinarily irritating whilst grieving prevents you from drowsing. Being continually upset, involved, and worn out can be crippling. The commonplace incidence of insomnia in people who are mourning need to only closing a quick even as. You must tell your health practitioner in case you preserve to have trouble falling asleep on time or feeling refreshed.

When Anger Turns into A Cycle

Many need to get over their loss and proceed healthily with their lives. The difficulty of this, even though, can also wonder a few. Grief has the capability to repeat itself. The mind's receptors can also on occasion get activated through mind of loss or a misplaced loved one. It can be quite challenging to transport on or "permit move." The grieving technique and those memories may additionally feed an addicted mood.

• Loneliness

The accompanying feelings of isolation is probably most of the maximum attempting elements of grief. If you shared a home with the deceased, you might now find your self on my own, probably for the initial time. It can be difficult to conform even if many buddies and circle of relatives are there. It is commonplace to miss someone certainly by their presence. You additionally would possibly lose hyperlinks to the human beings you know because of the deceased man or woman. Maybe they deliberate your life outside of work, or maybe you frolicked with their buddies and family lots. A demise may additionally pressure such ties.

After a dying, invitations may dwindle now and again. You can see that help and empathy generally tend to wane quickly after the funeral. It should seem as even though individuals close to you're now not going above and beyond. If you used to attend social gatherings together with your accomplice, circle of relatives, or buddies, you may locate it hard to do that anymore.

People do lose buddies whilst somebody passes away. Reaching out causes uncomfortable emotions; some humans can also even stop attempting altogether. Rejoining with others might be in particular tough if you are experiencing health troubles or have an impairment. Income, pensions, and economic affairs can all be impacted by a demise. It will be more tough to socialize as a end result.

Sorrow can go away you feeling alone even if surrounded by many humans. It may be tough for others to realize what you are managing whilst any person you have a unique connection with dies. The severity of the demise often makes this case worse. You may be the best character your age who has ever suffered this form of grief if you are younger. It could look like nobody else is to your scenario.

Everyone desires perfection to enhance with time; after they do not, the mourning man or woman may sense like there is whatever wrong with them. This can leave the mourning individual and the humans around them feeling helpless. It is vital to keep in thoughts that sorrow is a adventure. You will sometimes go through more extreme mourning reactions. That does no longer mean that your trip via unhappiness is made; as a substitute, you are passing through a despair.

You will in all likelihood continually mourn the loss in a sure way. However, there are a couple of techniques to deal with the isolation whilst persevering with your grieving technique and adjusting to the loss in your life.

• Fear

Online searches for signs and symptoms of worry provide a listing of feelings remarkably just like the ones of grief. Since it leaves you feeling so harassed, grief resembles terror. Consider how few matters we anticipate will give us a feeling of warranty in our life. We agree with that if we lead ethical lives, consume healthily, start looking after ourselves, and show love and attention to others, we can be blessed, and the human beings we care about may be kept secure. When the worst occurs, we surprise approximately our identities and where God is. What shall I do? What have to I do next? How can I continue? Even so, ought to I flow in any respect? It does appear pointless to care about nearly something, however not anything makes more sense. We lack self belief in our flesh and are uncertain who to accept as true with.

Because fear, in a manner, becomes our fact, grief seems like terror. We can construct our reality if we enjoy it and accept as true with it. We are there, however we aren't sure what we ought to do with it. Our darkest fears have come real. Fear and tension each evoke similar emotions. Fear is a recognizable chance, while anxiety is dread in the lack of a specific hazard. That does now not imply that the anxiety is justified. In reality, it is probably absolutely illogical and absurd.

Grief tends to concentrate at the past, however fear prefers to attention at the future. Since we're dubious of our capability to motive and decide matters a good way to not harm us greater, worry continues us from appearing. Fear paralyzes us and erodes our confidence in anyone and the entirety, even ourselves.

There is not any manner to maintain. We frequently withdraw from reality whilst we are terrified. To stay on this location feels more secure.

Fear is a healthful emotion. Fear can instruct us, as do all different feelings. If we permit it, it also can maintain us again. However, we're tougher and braver than we realise. There is a extra precedence some other place. Fear is merely the teacher.

• Anger

A common emotion is an anger. It is often used as a response to difficult or confrontational conditions. It won't typically come to mind while you take into account feeling sad because of a loss.

When a superb loss takes place, profound sorrow and other emotional reactions are frequently produced. You can revel in anger or irritability in conjunction with emotions of frustration, uncertainty, or shock.

Why did you enjoy this? How is this even possible? What is anticipated of you at the moment? When you are mourning, it is ordinary to feel irritated. You ought to take delivery of the right to witness this sensitive process absolutely.

Although sadness is every other important aspect of grief, it is able to additionally come over you concurrently as different emotions. Both rage and unhappiness are valid emotions. The wonderful fury felt whilst coping with a enormous loss is on occasion called "bereavement anger." Even if it looks like fury is the handiest feeling you're experiencing while experiencing anger for the duration of grief does not imply you are not sorry approximately your loss.

Not everybody goes thru those grieving ranges completely or within the genuine sequence. However, many humans's early and frequent stages of grief are recognised to include anger. Someone who is handling complicated grief can also endure lengthy-lasting wrath. Additionally, if anger predominates for the duration of your duration of sorrow, this will bring about protracted grief sickness.

You may want to turn out to be even greater dissatisfied after being irritated. It may want to make you experience awful approximately expressing your emotions in a way that your society would possibly don't forget wrong. Being harsh on oneself for having the feelings you do whilst you are dissatisfied should make you feel worst.

Like all other emotions, anger is a sense that can be felt and is first-class expressed moderately. Try instructing your self approximately the grieving cycle and discussing it with your family. This would possibly allow you to express your feelings with out frightening other people.

Another first rate alternative for letting your anger out is writing. You is probably capable of express your self through it with out virtually speakme to someone. To take care of this and other intense emotions, consider the usage of writing physical games.

• Guilt

Few emotions are extra hard to realize than the regret and guilt sensations which can follow the experience of grief. Regret and guilt are unpleasant feelings that often comply with other emotions. A person can also enjoy comfort that their beloved one is not any greater in ache and guilt over the initial sensation of remedy. Someone may also have anger approximately the occasions surrounding the demise, accompanied through guilt over the anger. The emotion that regularly is going along side other grief-related sentiments is guilt. One of the reasons which are so difficult to realise is this.

Additionally, it is simple to mix up the emotions of regret and guilt. If we attempt to realise this loss, we may additionally enjoy each of these feelings. Both of them can be extraordinarily scary and can bring about comparable conditions.

In times of grief, guilt may be a frequent but hard emotion. The reality is, there are a lot of things for which we can feel guilty. It is not vital for guilt to be logical to be actual. That implies we may additionally still feel guilty even after realizing it's miles unfounded.

To start with, we need to well known and recognize our guilt as one of the various regular responses that are an vital issue of the grieving technique. Second, we have to very well review it. How true is it? We regularly can also have exaggerated notions of what we're able to controlling or reaching. We can ponder if other people could decide us to be guilty. A commentary like that may help with perspective.

In other times, we'd need to take concrete action, consisting of writing a letter, talking to a vacant seat, or saying some thing at the cemetery. We may also need to investigate our ideals. Every faith or ideology recognizes the want to forgive others and ourselves. In mourning, guilt is a substantial weight. On the street to recuperation after loss, we do no longer have to bear guilt all the time.

It is regular to sense responsible or wish we had acted otherwise. We might want to be informed that we attempted our excellent, were exhausted or under pressure, or couldn't make it there in time. Just after truth, we either lose the impartiality vital to bear in mind the whole lot exactly because it changed into or forget what we did effectively.

There are approaches to get beyond regret if that's what you sense. It should involve putting your feelings in writing to the deceased individual in a letter. If there may be time, it is able to be discussing unresolved problems or unsolved difficulties with a terminally unwell man or woman.

3.2 Disturbed Professional Life

Many of us devote most of our day to work, where we may not have the nice friends notwithstanding spending most of our time with them. Although we might commit greater time to them than our partners, families, and co-workers, our encounters with them are regularly fleeting, and our conversations might not be in-depth. It makes experience then that the manifestation of grieving, that's hard to bring in spite of near buddies and family, is frequently suppressed at paintings; we are discussing the emotion of loss couldn't be allowed. Nobody is aware what to mention or do or what to avoid pronouncing or doing.

The grieving worker becomes a huge problem. Additionally, no matter the universality of grief and loss—sincerely every employee will come across them at a sure factor of their careers—those subjects are often unnoticed in the place of work, which may lead to disillusioned or complicated grief for the grieving parents in addition to lost productiveness and interruption of the administrative center for the employer.

While managers might also feel for his or her workforce, their number one responsibility is to get the venture finished. This may additionally war with offering sympathy or making an exception for a mourner's mediocre performance. Suppose a supervisor virtually desires to be sympathetic. In that case, they might experience powerless due to the fact they do no longer recognize how to speak to grieving workers or because senior control has no longer supported or directed them, leaving them with none power, guidelines, or policies to intrude. As a result, they may at great ignore a grieving colleague or be pressured to put into effect disciplinary measures, together with delaying a improve because of allegedly bad performance.

Coworkers once in a while enjoy challenge or resentment over a employee's declining potential to carry out their responsibilities and the requirement to jump in and fill the void despite their compassion for a bereaved colleague.

Tasks and obligations can be not noted whilst grieving to recognition on dealing with the loss. Employers should have a activity executed, and the sufferer nevertheless wishes to go to paintings. The bereaved man or woman's coworkers couldn't comprehend why they're now not doing what they ought to be, why they are no longer carrying out their responsibilities, why the extent in their work has reduced, or why they appearance fed up in the assignment at hand.

The workplace struggles to balance assisting grieving employees and ensuring production. Typically, people use clock or agenda time to decide how lengthy it's miles suitable for the individual to be less powerful. Coworkers entreated to help out to ease the load on grieving personnel are affected. Their productivity may then go through, which might cause hatred. A institution that can be empathetic to dropping however is beaten by means of the preference to finish a project may additionally come to be demoralized because of the domino effect it is able to reason.

Social folks who have interaction one-on-one with mourning humans can help by using offering them aid, recommendation, and statistics about available neighborhood resources ought to they require additional help. However, they can also resource geared especially towards work-related troubles. For instance, they are able to "assist the people in processing what they require and how to express that to their managers and coworkers."

three.Three Compromised Health

It is startling how physically taxing grieving may be. Your heart hurts so awful. You recollect some thing that makes your belly turn or sends a shiver down your backbone. Sometimes you could rarely nod off because your body is so charged with electricity that it causes your heart and brain to race. Sometimes you're so exhausted which you nod off right away. The following morning, you wake up, still feeling worn out, and spend most of the week in mattress.

Sleep Issues

You might also battle to get the everyday rest your frame and thoughts require in case you are grieving. You will have problems falling asleep, frequent middle of the night awakenings, or maybe immoderate sleep. Sleeping properly may be beneficial. Go to sleep, arise at the identical time every day, and relax before bed with some thing calming like a shower, a unique, or respiration sports.

Numerous research studies have shown that grieving individuals have problem falling and preserving asleep. Whether the man or woman become depressed or now not, this become the state of affairs. People who are grieving regularly experience sleep disturbances, that could negatively have an effect on their physical and emotional fitness.

Fatigue

Grief's emotional toll can sap your electricity. Even in case you do not feel like consuming, eat sufficient to keep your energy. Exercise is also vital; even a short walk might be useful. Maintaining relationships with loved ones is likewise beneficial. Additionally, a aid institution or a mental fitness professional should provide you with a sense of network and techniques for purchasing through your sorrow.

Compromised Immune System

Your body's defense against pathogens is furnished with the aid of your immune gadget, a complicated system of cells, organs, and organs. It defends your body from out of doors intruders which can make you unwell. An occasion that is habitually by way of grief after the loss of life of a near relative has more than one results on physical and intellectual health, which leads to a faded immune gadget. Diseases and illnesses may result from a compromised immune system.

Inflammation

Your frame's tissues make bigger due to your immune system reacting to what it perceives as a risk. Cardiovascular sickness, osteoarthritis, weight problems, asthma, and most cancers can be affected. There is records that indicates irritation and grief are associated, and a few research shows the infection worsens the more profound the grief. You can control it via getting sufficient exercise and consuming nicely.

Digestion

You would possibly forestall eating often or binge while you are grieving. Hormone ranges can also give you the flu or aggravate your intestine and other parts of your digestive system. You can get ulcers, irritable bowel diarrhea, constipation, and abdominal cramps. Your health practitioner can help you in locating treatments in case you are experiencing persistent stomach troubles.

The emotional and bodily additives of mourning are connected. The same structures system physical and psychological stress within the frame, and both sorts can comfortably cause the nervous system to become energetic. High adrenalin and coronary heart rate added on by means of continual stress can be a factor in lengthy-term medical issues. Depression is a consequence of grieving rather than a natural detail of it. Understanding depression's symptoms are crucial due to the fact they increase the chance of fitness problems related to grieving and are regularly dealt with to relieve.

According to analyze, rumination, or constantly unsightly, self-targeted thought, is a method for warding off troubles. Ruminators consciousness on bad cloth that is more dangerous than the painful realities they need to avoid, diverting attention away from them. Depression has a strong affiliation with this manner of thinking. The herbal capacities of the thoughts and physique to assimilate new truths and heal are blocked with the aid of ruminating and different avoidance behaviors that use power.

three.Four Loss Grief Trauma is Dangerous

Losing a beloved one, going thru a awful incident, or seeing others revel in misfortune can be hard and emotionally arduous. You may even believe that your melancholy sentiments will constantly be there. Luckily, there are effective techniques for processing your feelings and transferring on at the same time as paying admire to a misplaced cherished one or horrible occasion.

Psychological trauma is a person's emotional response to a frightful, horrifying, or scary event or a sequence of events. Unexpected worrying conditions can bring about extreme stress beyond your potential to deal with them. Trauma can often reason you to impeach your beliefs concerning life, your feeling of control, your feel of protection, and self belief in different human beings. Anxiety and terror might end result from losing those middle sentiments of safety and faith. Even your beliefs may be referred to as into query in case you experience that the arena is risky and unpredictable. Post-annoying strain disorder and lengthy-time period mental trauma can also end result from extreme strain. Any mental trauma can make it tough if you want to hold a courting, perform daily responsibilities, and experience existence.

Frequently happening catastrophes may lead to "compassion fatigue" and "psychic numbing," wherein the thoughts dissociates emotions from grieving-associated thoughts. At first, you might not sense anything, but days or even months in the past, numerous feelings might unexpectedly sweep over you. Do now not experience terrible if you address trauma extra slowly than others or in case you absorb the loss in another way. The grieving method you're going through, and your emotions are unique to you. The effective aspect Although going thru horrible experiences and managing sorrow is difficult and draining; the experience can help you in becoming more potent and growing your resilience. You will conquer this tough moment, and assistance is available.

Grief is a painful but inevitable element of lifestyles. When an extended dating has ended, while we lose a cherished one, or when we go through different styles of loss, we grieve. A loss is usually anticipated or foreseeable, like dropping an elderly discern to a disease. The ordinary mourning system can be interrupted, made worse, and prolonged when the loss of life is unanticipated given that stress and grief occur in those conditions. A intellectual fitness expert's counseling or different forms of professional useful resource are often essential for traumatic grief recovery.

Chapter 9: A Comprehensive Grief Journey – A Five-Step Handling

When the main purpose is to learn how to tackle the difficulty of loss and grief, it's far essential to understand the difficulty from the very begin. The same rule have to be implemented to complex troubles like the grief of loss and their negative affects. When you absolutely recognize the difficulty, you will most effective be capable of tackle it nicely.

2.1 Acknowledging your Grief is the First Step

Learning greater about the mourning system might be useful in case you or a close one is experiencing a loss. Here, we can go through the 5 degrees of grief and a few tips for assisting someone mourning a loss or separation.

It is crucial to remember that everyone's grief system is unique and is probably complicated. You won't comply with those directions flawlessly, or you would possibly enjoy new emotions after you accept as true with you have got handed and are thru the grief tiers. You might start to recover from a loss by using permitting yourself to sense disappointment on your way.

Elisabeth Kübler-Ross, a psychiatrist, devised the "five Stages of Grief" speculation. It means that we enjoy 5 distinctive stages after dropping a loved one.

• Denial

Rejection aids us in lessening the intense grief of loss during the initial tiers of the mourning system. We try to endure emotional struggling even as we come to acknowledge the fact of our grief. It is probably difficult to simply accept their passing if we've got closing spoken to a key discern in our lives inside the closing week or even an afternoon.

At this factor in the mourning manner, our world has totally modified. Our minds might also want a while to get used to our new international. When someone close to us passes away, we often suppose returned on the activities we had and war with a way to move on without them.

There is much data to have a look at and tough photographs to technique. Denial makes an effort to gradual down the manner and guide us thru it step-through-step in place of take the risk of turning into crushed with emotion.

• Anger

Anger is the second degree of grieving. We are probable in exquisite emotional ache as we battle to deal with a brand-new reality. There are more than one things to do not forget that we may want to feel like rage gives us a way to specific our emotions.

Remember that rage does now not want us to be mainly exposed. It may, although, seem more culturally desirable than to acknowledge our worry. Anger shall we us specific our emotions with out traumatic about being judged or rejected.

We often enjoy anger as the first feeling we launch after experiencing a loss. As a result, we should feel on my own in our stories. Additionally, it could make us appear remote to people while we need their help, closeness, and reassurance.

• Bargaining

It is commonplace to have such desperation even as handling loss that you might be willing to try whatever to reduce the struggling. To trade the instances at some stage in this section of grief, you may offer to take action in alternate for comfort from the discomfort you are experiencing.

When we start to negotiate, we regularly deal with our demands to a higher authority or to something more effective than ourselves that is probably capable of have an effect on a distinct final results. We bargain out of a sense of powerlessness as it makes what appears so out of our manipulate more potential. When we bargain, we often dwell on our shortcomings or regrets. When we replicate on our relationships with the man or woman we are losing, we are able to see all the instances when we felt distant from them or probable harm them.

It is normal to assume lower back on times whilst we would have spoken something we surely did now not mean and needed we could change how we behaved. We also from time to time count on that we would now not be in this kind of horrible emotional scenario proper now if occasions transpired in another way.

• Depression

There comes the factor in the levels of grief while our mind cool down, and we gradually remember the truth of our current occasions. We are confronted with the situation and experience like negotiation is no more an alternative.

We start to enjoy the demise of our beloved one extra intensely in the course of this degree of grief. Our tension begins to reduce, the mental haze begins to lift, and the loss turns into more tangible and inevitable.

As the unhappiness intensifies, we have a tendency to withdraw. We can discover that we withdraw, are less pleasant, and communicate to others less concerning what we are experiencing. Even whilst sadness after a loved one's demise can be keeping apart, it's miles a fairly normal step of the grief system.

• Acceptance

Acceptance is the last of all stages of grief. We do not forestall feeling the grief of loss while we reach a point of acceptance. Rather, we are not preventing against the statistics of our instances or looking to trade them.

In this degree, sadness and sorrow are nevertheless feasible. However, all through this stage of the grieving system, the emotional coping mechanisms of denial, negotiation, and rage are less probable to exist.

In wellknown, if we are not on the recognition level, we resist or ignore statistics come what may. We may begin to sleep more. The attention of our interest may additionally shift to our emotions of gloom or worrisome mind, deflecting from outside pressures. We can also move toward drugs or alcohol to get away or detach from fact. To prevent experiencing misery, we may additionally attention on our duties, tasks, or other human beings's wishes.

Acceptance does not mean that one is incapable of feeling pain, sorrow, or tragedy. It does not imply that you approve of what is taking area. It involves spotting what you're battling, maintaining your choice to achieve this, and realigning yourself with the prevailing circumstances. It includes keeping off getting stuck or shifting past different stages of being stuck. Being aware and having a curious, open attitude can be quite beneficial.

Rarely do the ranges development in a straight line. Mood swings and changes in ideas, ideals, and behaviors are commonplace. When circumstances appear so unpleasant, it could be challenging to maintain reputation. If you experience careworn, you aren't required to undergo sorrow, loss, or trauma alone. The counseling centers can offer culturally-sensitive guide and path through the grieving technique.

2.2 Express Yourself Completely

Usually, talking about your unhappiness will not be enough after a expensive one, regardless of whether or not they handed away suddenly or spent several months in healthcare. Perhaps you aren't saying the whole lot you meant to say with your comments. Or they fail to explicit how deeply you feel correct. This is why conducting inventive expression is a vital factor of human existence and a remarkable technique to deal with any poor feelings you will be experiencing, specifically during tough times like loss. For many people, enticing inside the expression of self can assist in bringing complicated, ingrained sentiments to the surface.

You may also need to reflect onconsideration on starting a innovative endeavor as 1/2 of your grieving manner. Painting is regularly the primary thing that involves mind for maximum folks, however you're underneath no want to begin painting. There are diverse approaches to apply creativity to explicit your self and find out what lies beyond the surface.

We all have skilled the sensation of being speechless. There can be some things you absolutely cannot explicit after accompanying a cherished one through intensive care. By expressing yourself creatively, you can come to be extra aware of your feelings. You can take some time at some point of the artistic thinking to mirror to your feelings, deeds, attitudes, and behaviors. If you spend time investigating it, you may be blind to something occurring within.

A huge variety of emotions may be induced by way of grief. Some of those feelings would possibly even give you tension or fear. Using your creativity, you could exhibit yourself accurately at the same time as handling loss. When you provoke, no one else is required to be present until you need them to. It is a moment when you have the option of going by myself to research your innermost mind and feelings thoughtfully. Even if the feelings that floor are unpleasant, it's far higher to allow them to out than to keep them bottled up interior, awaiting an possibility to burst. Your activity is as private as you select it to be.

Since the one that you love's incurable analysis, you have been on a rollercoaster.

It shook your world when they surpassed away. Things that once felt strong and solid should now appear risky and unsure. Depending on how extreme the loss turned into, it could appear as though the whole lot changed into spinning out of manipulate. By growing a innovative exercise, you open up the opportunity of having some have an impact on over just one place of your existence. You are the boss, and also you set the rules. Throughout the procedure, inventiveness could prove to be a honest companion and a manner to maintain oneself whilst faced with uncertainty and struggling.

Some humans will determine to exhibit their creativity on my own. Others will capture the risk to participate in institution innovative expression. You may accomplice with other artists experiencing loss if you pick to color. If you write approximately grief, you might be a part of a poetry writing organization. You are never on my own in your journey; many people deal with loss differently. You may meet a sympathetic character in a class who will aid you while grieving.

Most humans lose a loved one by the time they are in their senior yr of excessive college. It takes experiencing grief to recognize the concept of it. Each man or woman's reaction to grief is particular, depending on their relationship with the deceased and other factors. Physiological reaction to the energy of feelings felt is one of the few things that continuously arise throughout mourning, even though it is a very individualized method.

Even if one is blind to their sentiments, everyone stories them bodily. We can select to pay attention and use our know-how to hyperlink the messages our bodies send us all the time. Our our bodies, for instance, alert us whenever we're ravenous or want to sleep. Similarly, the burden in our chest may also sign a cherished one's forthcoming birthday, which has exceeded away. Or the difficulty in speakme is mirrored within the compression of the throat. Given the depth of our emotions at some stage in mourning, it makes experience that our bodies might require a way to explicit themselves.

Journaling is a attempted-and-trusted approach of coming across the way you experience because it offers you the distance and time to do it privately. Having the words to deliver your innermost thoughts might assist you higher recognize your self, but you do no longer need to proportion them with each person except you pick out to.

No one will care if you do not assume you are a terrific creator. Start easy, which includes with what you probably did or who you had spoken to that day if you sense self-aware.

Also, by no means be scared to use your creativeness. Use various colored pens, doodles, caricature, and rip aside pages. There is no right or incorrect manner to write down in a journal; you are loose to do as you want. One of the maximum annoying elements of grieving is which you can't communicate to handiest one character you would love to speak to. A message to the one you love, even if you know they'll no longer be able to see it, would possibly help you procedure your emotions on their passing and reveal any unstated troubles that are affecting you.

Another method is to put in writing letters to other individuals. Try writing a letter first if you are having problem communicating your feelings to a pal or member of your own family. You aren't required to ship the letter; you may just use it to remind your self of your intentions.

2.Three Focus on Reconnecting (Putting Pieces Together Again)

The loss of a better one is in no way simple. You can experience isolated, forget your traditional habitual, or find which you no longer discover specific sports fun. Staying in may additionally seem like a far easier route than the preparations you made with friends. Shutting out the arena can be a better choice, but if this manner of life persists for too lengthy, there'll not be any recovery. How are we able to keep taking part in things that please us, mainly when we do no longer suppose as we will? How are we able to re-interact with lifestyles in potential steps?

The daily hassles and concerns of the out of doors global are simpler to lose your self in than ever. Our attention is continuously directed faraway from ourselves and towards such things as paintings, relationships, and errands. For many of us, it's far a never-ending battle to delight people or to behave in a manner that we accept as true with is needed to win their love, regard, or popularity.

You are not required to accept less than capable of being, sharing, giving, or growing. You can understand your abilities and analyze what surely motivates you when you re-establish contact with yourself. The more you are aware about this, the greater you may be able to make a contribution to the world and the way others see you. Now is the suitable time to test what motivates you. What offers you the greatest experience of existence? Your lifestyles's work.

When turned into the ultimate time I turned into happiest? What do I do once I am feeling most like myself? When nobody else is there, how do I talk with myself? It is your present to me. Your actual self. The secret to getting back in touch with oneself.

Finding your task is not always truthful. Humans get into disempowering behaviors that preserve us in a never-ending cycle of failure. We have restrictive thoughts about what we're able to in existence. We allow society or our family to set expectancies on us with the aid of adhering to a pattern for pleasure that we did no longer create.

Your present might be associated with helping or doing desirable worldwide in case you need to contribute. If you yearn for importance or connection, circle of relatives and buddies are possibly vital parts of your life's purpose. You can start mastering a way to re-connect to yourself after you become aware of your finest human need.

Believing that you do not should have your desires addressed consequences from your restricting ideals. Stop always putting others earlier than your self and forgetting to refill your cup. Once you have decided what you need, satisfy it. Spend a while being concerned for your self. Request what you need from others. You may additionally make a contribution extra from the vicinity of achievement by way of being your real self.

Investigate and choose the pleasant possibilities as you gradually reenter day by day lifestyles, in search of tiny opportunities to engage. This could be creating a short telephone name to a buddy, meeting for an hour-long cup of espresso, or going to lunch or the movies. When it involves recuperation, no effort is too modest; go your own pace.

Embrace your emotions. The more poor emotions that we usually need to keep away from are particularly erratic whilst someone is grieving. Because they may be so hefty, it will take all of your energy to get off the bed a few days. Do now not berate yourself in case you want to vacation from paintings for a couple of hours or spend the day in mattress. Recognize your barriers, however do not be embarrassed by means of them.

Be ambitious on your outreach to others. Tell your loved ones that you're going thru a grieving technique and might not be the equal man or woman you were as soon as, but that you want their agency and guide. Even in case you decline their invites the first few times, do now not be scared to ask buddies to touch on you now and again and to hold doing so.

Understanding that grieving is a process as opposed to an event is crucial. It alters who we are, how we view the world, and the way we engage with others. Grief, however, does not cease while we're required to maintain our ordinary duties, which includes work, education, and circle of relatives care. As you resume your ordinary sports, bear in mind to offer your self area and time to your grieving in addition to a number of the stuff you used to love doing earlier than your loss, which permit you to feel just a little bit very just like yourself.